Pilates

For Core Strength

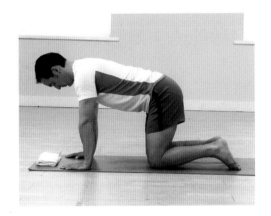

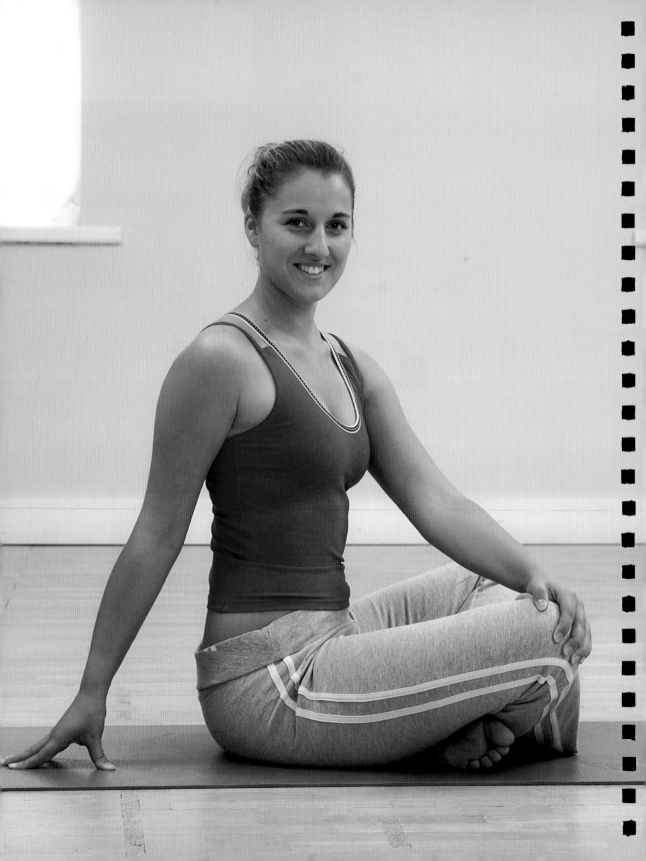

Pilates
For Core Strength

A STEP-BY-STEP GUIDE

IMPROVE CORE STRENGTH AND STABILITY

30-MINUTE WORKOUTS

Sandie Keane

Main Street
A division of Sterling Publishing Co., Inc.
New York

Library of Congress Cataloging-in-Publication Data Available

10 9 8 7 6 5 4 3 2 1

Published by Main Street a division of Sterling Publishing Co., Inc.
387 Park Avenue South, New York, NY 10016
© 2005 by PRC Publishing
An imprint of **Chrysalis** Books Group plc

Distributed in Canada by Sterling Publishing
c/o Canadian Manda Group, 165 Dufferin Street
Toronto, Ontario, Canada M6K 3H6

Printed in China

1 4027 1971 X

The exercise programs described in this book are based on well-established
practices proven to be effective for over-all health and fitness, but they are
not a substitute for personalized advice from a qualified practitioner. Always
consult with a qualified health care professional in matters relating to your
health before beginning this or any exercise program. This is especially
important if you are pregnant or nursing, if you are elderly, or if you have
any chronic or recurring medical condition. As with any exercise program,
if at any point during your workout you begin to feel faint, dizzy, or have
physical discomfort, you should stop immediately and consult a physician.

The purpose of this book is to educate and is sold with the
understanding that the author and the publisher shall have neither liability
nor responsibility for any injury caused or alleged to be caused directly
or indirectly by the information contained in this book.

Contents

Introduction

Acquiring balance and equilibrium in one's body takes a little time and effort, but with the understanding that "less is more," it is achievable. Pilates offers you a gentle but powerful approach to achieving your natural potential for optimal strength, flexibility, and stamina. It could be said that Pilates is unique in its delivery as it can be personalized for specific medical conditions and posture types.

The Pilates method is a body conditioning exercise therapy, targeting the deep postural muscles to achieve core stability and strength with improved muscle balance. It involves the re-alignment of the spine to its optimum position with gentle stretching and strengthening movements. Pilates exercises are particularly recommended for those who suffer from chronic neck or back pain, postural problems, sports injuries, osteoporosis, arthritis, stress-related illnesses, M.E., and many other conditions. It is a safe, effective way of exercising, as you are encouraged to execute the moves slowly and within your own range of movement, so it falls within everyone's capabilities from the top athlete looking to enhance their performance and avoid the risk of injury, to clients who have never exercised much before.

Back pain is epidemic in America. It costs over $4 billion each year and, aside from the common cold, keeps more people away from work than any other single cause. Medical studies suggest that over 26 million people in the U.S.A. die each year due to lack of physical activity. Diverse evidence from many cultures show that sitting has been associated with: back pain, fatigue, varicose veins, stress, problems with the diaphragm, circulation, digestion, and colonic problems to name but a few. The answer lies in re-educating the body to move the way it was designed. Simply by using the body properly, "autonomous" sitting can be regained. Pilates can help to achieve this.

Over the years the principles associated with Pilates have been tried and tested by a variety of professions and toward the end of the twentieth century it was acknowledged by the medical profession that Pilates based exercises were extremely beneficial in the correction of spinal alignment and for joint rehabilitation. It is now practiced worldwide by osteopaths and physiotherapists. The medical profession will now, where appropriate, refer patients to a Pilates practitioner so they can learn how to integrate it into their daily life. This is because the principles can be incorporated when standing, sitting, lifting, and performing household chores. It is more than an exercise program, it is a lifestyle.

Joseph Pilates

Joseph Pilates was born in 1880 in Germany. He was a sickly child, but born with a determination to overcome his physical frailties. He studied many exercise disciplines such as yoga, gymnastics, various other sports, even circus training. He subsequently became an accomplished skier, diver, gymnast, and boxer. Practicing his techniques on himself and others he soon developed an exercise philosophy which combined strength, flexibility, and stamina. With his unique knowledge and understanding of the body, the series of exercises he

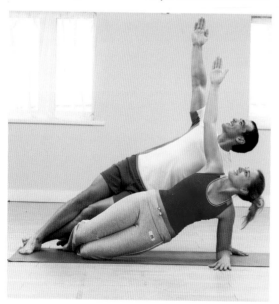

developed are still being practiced today. There are many variations relating to the principles of Pilates ranging from those that he himself pioneered in the early 1900s to the contemporary approach that incorporates a modern understanding of fitness, anatomy, and biomechanics. The essential principles however have over the years been simplified, so that anybody of any age, aptitude, or fitness level can benefit. Pilates is more than a passing exercise trend. Many of our top sportsmen and athletes use Pilates regularly in their training regimes, but it is now increasingly popular with older clients, particularly those of retirement age. Post-natal women are encouraged to include these exercises after childbirth, when they are looking to re strengthen their abdominal muscles and restore body shape. It has of course attracted many celebrities who now swear by this method. Jennifer Aniston, Courtney Cox, Gwyneth Paltrow, Rod Stewart, Sarah Jessica Parker, Hugh Grant, and Uma Thurman, to name but a few, are among the stars who practice Pilates.

Pilates, after many years of research, came to the conclusion that if we concentrated on moving slowly and effortlessly while maintaining correct alignment, the results were profound in the improvement of core strength, flexibility, posture, and balance. With these key components in place, the added benefits that presented themselves were that bone density remained steady, which helps to ward off increased risk of osteoporosis, and synovial fluid increased around the joints helping to fight against joint stiffness.

It appears that the only side effects from Pilates, if executed correctly, are improved posture, inner strength, toned muscles, and relief from tension and stress.

Inspiration from the East

Having studied the Eastern disciplines, Pilates incorporated the interaction of mind and body, placing great emphasis on the way we breathe and how our breathing could aid or distort movement. Because your mind is required to engage with your body to perform the movements correctly, you experience a new awareness of muscle function and control.

With the emphasis on breath and body awareness, the capacity in mental focus deepens to a degree where the psychological changes have been proven to be positive.

With the popularity of Pilates growing, classes are on the increase. Since its commercial arrival in the late 1990s, it has revolutionized the exercise and fitness industry following years of high impact, go for the burn workouts. The overall appeal of a slower more sensible approach has been welcomed by many. A program that you can look forward to, one that engages you and leaves you refreshed, alert, and with a feeling of physical and mental well-being.

The demand however for qualified teachers has proved problematic. The concern turns to the fitness clubs where teachers are put through fast track courses to supply the demand from the public. Many of these courses unfortunately produce less than adequately qualified teachers, which poses a dilemma for the medical profession who refer patients to such classes for rehabilitation only to find that the level of the class exceeds the abilities of those attending.

Competently trained and knowledgeable practitioners are an essential element in realizing someone's potential. These practitioners have undergone many hours of training and with some many years of study, when you find one they are invaluable. There are many around now who have specialized in this field.

The exercises in this book are safe for the beginner. Books and videos are exceptionally good for reference but they cannot take the place of learning one-on-one with a qualified teacher. Use the more advanced exercises with discretion and if in doubt look for advice from a qualified Pilates practitioner or consult your doctor. Some of the exercises may be unsuitable for your state of health and therefore need to be avoided. A postural analysis and medical questionnaire should be undertaken if you ever commence a group session.

What Do You Achieve From Pilates?

It is agreed by all organizations that the principles listed below all adhere to the Pilates method. When introducing these principles at the beginning it can be quite daunting so although they are integral to the practice many of them are achieved while working through the five basic principles detailed further on.

Relaxation: This is very important when starting Pilates. Learning to relax and recognize areas of tension that need releasing.

Concentration: It is the mind itself that builds the body and that all important connection between mind and body comes with concentration.

Alignment: Proper alignment is the key to good posture. Learning to feel where every part of the body is at any one time is explained and outlined in the five basic principles.

Breathing: Natural, conscious breathing patterns coordinated with movement helps to activate muscles and keep you focused.

Centering: Focusing on the muscles of the pelvic floor and deep abdominals develops a strong core and enables the rest of the body to function efficiently. All action initiates from the center and flows outward to the extremities.

Coordination: When combining two or three movements we go through the phases of learning. We start with the "cognitive stage," proceed to the "motor stage," before we reach the "automatic phase." This takes practice but achieves results.

Fluidity: Pilates requires smooth, continuous movement, which is effortless but strong.

Stamina: Endurance is built up slowly, which challenges strength and stability.

There are an number of mnemonics you can use to remember Pilates, in fact you can make up your own from this list.

P	**Posture, Precision, Poise, Personal, Proficient, Practical, Powerful, Profound**
I	**Intense, Informative, Intelligent, Internal, Improvement**
L	**Learning, Lengthening, Leisurely, Loosening, Litheness, Lasting, Longevity, Lifestyle**
A	**Ability, Aptitude, Agility, Appreciation, Activity Accredited, Athletic, Awareness, Alignment**
T	**Thorough, Thinking, Training, Total, True, Tone, Transverse Abdominus**
E	**Efficient, Educational, Easy, Enjoyable, Equilibrium, Experience Established, Elongating, Everlasting, Elastic, Energy, Expanding**
S	**Stability, Slow, Strength, Slender, Sequential, Suppleness Synchronisation, Stamina**

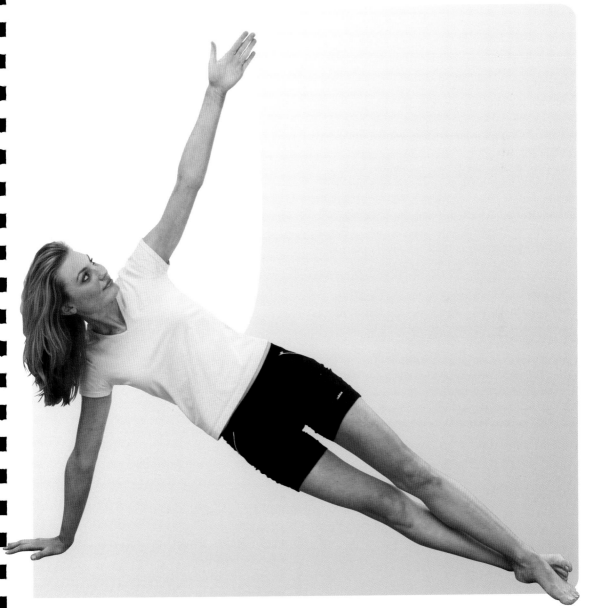

Self-Postural Analysis

It is a good idea to take a look at your posture, which will help you when choosing a program that will benefit you most. Follow these simple guidelines to check your own posture. If you can persuade someone to help you then it will make things easier but it can be done on your own. Whatever your posture may be at this present time, you need to understand the basic language used to help get into better alignment. No matter how fit you are, understanding the basic principles are the key to the profound results Pilates can offer. Setting up your position is the most important thing when learning the basics. There is really no point in learning an exercise if your posture is out of alignment before you begin.

The exercises given in this book are shown at different levels. If you are unable to attend a class or get private tuition for a short time then please take care with the progressive exercises. The rule of thumb is, if you are struggling or tension is presenting itself then the level is too strong for you at that time. Remember less is more.

You will need a full-length mirror and be able to see your shape so wear something tight fitting, such as a swimsuit. Stand in front of the mirror and adopt your normal stance.

Imagine you are standing in the middle of a clock face facing 12 o'clock. Write down what you see on the self analysis sheet and come back to it in a couple of month's time to see how things have changed. Look at the analysis sheet that follows and see how you shape up.

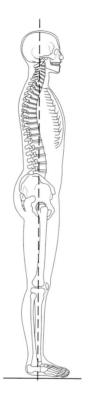

An example of optimal posture with the plumb line running through the center of the body.

Date:

Feet
Standing in the middle of your imaginary clock face, look at your feet in the mirror.
Where are they pointing?
Draw their position on the clock.

Knees
Where are your knees pointing?
- Level ☐
- Left higher than right/right higher than left ☐
- Facing forward ☐
- Left knee turned in/right knee turned in/both knees turned in ☐

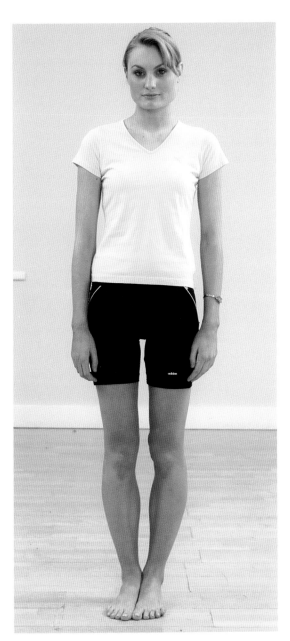

Here the feet both point to around 12:05 on an imaginary clock and the knees are noticeably turned in especially the left.

Hip bones

Place your middle fingers on the bones at the front of your body commonly known as your hip bones.

Then look at your fingers.
Are they?
• Level ☐
• Left finger higher than right/right finger ☐
higher than left

In the picture (left) notice the gap between her left arm and her body and the gap between her right arm and body. This indicates that the hips are not sitting level and that the right side is slightly higher than the left.

Look at the gaps that you have, they should be the same if you have good alignment.

Rib cage

Place your hands on your rib cage and find the bottom of the ribs with one finger. (They will be much lower than you think.) Look at your fingers in the mirror.

Are they?

• Level? ☐
• Left side higher than right/right side ☐
higher than left?

Shoulders

Look at your shoulders to see if they sit:
• Level ☐
• Left side higher than right/right side higher ☐
than left

If you look at the picture (left) you will notice that one shoulder sits higher than the other.

Head

Where does your head sit on your shoulders?
• Centrally ☐
• Tipped to the left/right ☐

11

If you have someone to help you, get your helper to view you from the side or ask them to take a photograph of you and place an imaginary plumb line through the body. The pictures (below) show a kyphotic/flatback posture, typically characterized by rounded shoulders.

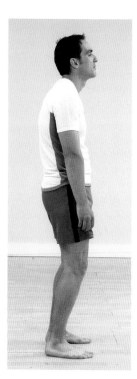 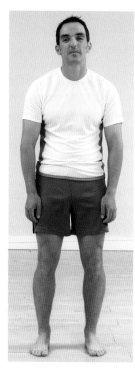

Kyphotic/flatback posture from the side.

Kyphotic/flatback posture from the front

Side

Where does your head sit?
- Centrally ☐
- Further forward/back of the line ☐

What is your neck length?
- Short ☐
- Long ☐

Where do your arms sit?
- Centrally (middle finger down seam of your clothes at the side) ☐
- Forward ☐

Is your upper back?
- Flat ☐
- Rounded ☐

Is your lower back?
- Flat ☐
- Over arching ☐

Are your knees?
- Bent slightly forward ☐
- Hyperextended (bent backward) ☐

Back/front

Ask your helper again to view you from both the front and back or take photographs as an accurate record of your posture.

Is your head sitting on your shoulders?
- Centrally ☐
- To the left/right ☐

Are your shoulders?
- Level ☐
- Left/right higher ☐

Are the creases in the back of your knees level?
- Yes ☐
- No ☐

Are your ankles?
- Straight ☐
- Left/right toward center (dropped arches) ☐

Once you have completed your postural analysis you can then look to see what posture type you fall into. We never fall into just one, it will be a bit of a mixture but you will be able to put yourself into one or two easily.

Pilates is a Personal Thing

Everyone's posture is determined by their genetics, lifestyle, activity, and emotions. If you look at a foetus in the womb the spine is one shape; we are born with a rounded spine. The "s" shape develops during the early stages of our growth giving us our kyphotic and lordotic curves. These curves are important to maintain as they absorb impact when we walk, run, or jump. If these curves are not present then the shock waves traveling up from our feet would go straight to the head.

As we grow our muscles develop, supporting the skeleton as it moves. During childhood the number of movement patterns we performed throughout one day was infinite. This allowed the body to be nourished constantly and consequently we could move in all kinds of ways without causing ourselves any damage. Unfortunately as we get older, our lifestyles and recreation become more sedentary and our movement patterns are reduced even though our bodies are capable of flexibility. By the time we reach our 20s most of us have reduced our patterns to sitting, standing and lying only. This is down to our lifestyles inhibiting our natural movement patterns. The use of the car and labor saving devices limit our physical activity.

In these cases the result is prolonged alteration of the natural curves of the spine and stress will be placed on the joints causing eventual pain. This is commonly described as repetitive strain syndrome. In an optimal posture the forces of gravity should be evenly distributed through the body with the muscles being at their optimal length and strength in order to support the skeleton efficiently.

If we had an ideal posture, then our skeletal system would be supported by our deep postural stabilizing muscles. We would then have our movement muscles all working at their optimum strength and flexibility in order to move us effortlessly. If all of our muscles and joints were working in harmony we would move, according to Joseph Pilates, "like the sound of a finely tuned orchestra." Every part playing efficiently and effectively for the purpose it was intended.

Wouldn't that be nice if we all had perfect posture? But our bodies undertake days, months, and years of strain and abuse resulting from our habits.

When you first look at changing your posture then you have to look at what posture type you fall into. Unfortunately we never fall into just one type of posture as one can be the cause of another. You need to look generally at where you need to either lengthen short muscles or strengthen weak ones in order to restore optimal alignment.

If you spend your working hours seated or standing then your movement patterns will be directly affected due to sustained positions and repetitive movements. Therefore your working environment plays a huge role in how you hold yourself.

Let us look at the four main posture types to give you an idea of which type you may fall into:

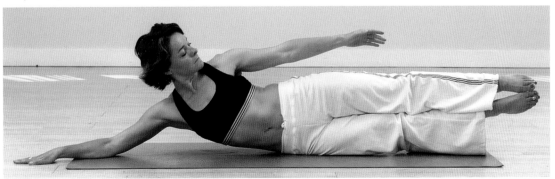

Posture Types

LORDOTIC

The lordotic posture is the type you see in young gymnasts. It is also a posture seen in pregnant women and men with a beer belly due to the extra weight being carried in front. If you look at the picture below, notice that the abdominals are lengthened and the lower back is tight, which places excessive stress on the lumbar discs, causing the muscles to be over active. We often wrongly recruit the lumbar muscles when carrying or lifting heavy objects, placing more stress than is already present.

For example, when carrying heavy shopping we should be recruiting the shoulder and core stabilizers rather then relying on the lumbar extensors to support the spine. This is a common trait in those who are lordotic, creating unnecessary tension in the lower back which causes stiffness and immobility in that area. This can prove difficult to correct initially. The excessive curve which is present in a lordotic posture is there because the pelvis is being held in an anterior tilt where the hip bones are forward of the pubic bone. This position of the pelvis also causes the hip flexors to shorten and the hamstrings to be lengthened. Mobility exercises will help considerably in helping to correct these problems but care needs to be taken in executing movement in the lower back due to the probable stiffness. The spine needs to be encouraged to move slowly and gently to avoid any forced error of movement. Less is more.

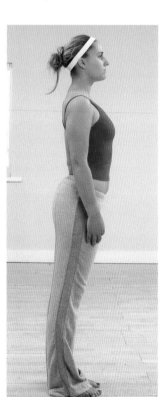

Problems
- Weak gluteals (buttocks)
- Over active hamstrings
- Short hip flexors
- Weak abdominals

Solutions
- Strengthen abdominals and gluteals (buttocks)
- Increase segmental control of the spine to reduce lordosis and increase mobility
- Lengthen hip flexors
- Stretch back extensors

Exercises
- Supine set position
- Pelvic tilts
- Knee drops
- Hamstring stretch
- Shoulder bridge
- Abdominal preparation
- Seated "c" curve
- Seated spine twist
- All fours: cat pedals, cat's tail
- Shell stretch
- Hip flexor stretch
- Arm floats
- Monkey squat

KYPHOTIC

Kyphosis is the posture that has the round-shouldered appearance. It is seen mainly in those who have sedentary jobs, such as office workers and those who sit all day at a computer or drive for a living. Sitting causes major postural imbalances in the spine and affects the length, strength, and stamina in certain muscles.

For example, when your body is sitting in a chair all day the muscles that should be supporting you are actually inhibited. The buttocks, our biggest muscle in the body, can very often be our weakest. The leg muscles are also inhibited when sitting as they too are being supported but they are also being kept in a bent position for long periods which can cause the hamstrings in the back of the legs to shorten and the quads at the front of the legs to lengthen. All are inactive while sitting so have a tendency to be weak. We then have to accept that the muscles in the ankles and feet are not taking any weight all day so they too become weaker. Lastly the position of the head is never at its optimal position when sitting especially at a computer when you're constantly looking down at the keyboard then up at the screen, the neck muscles work extremely hard to support the head which tends to poke forward shortening the neck extensors at the back of the neck and lengthening the neck flexors which are at the front.

Slumping is common when sitting and this is contributory to many digestive problems as well as muscular imbalances. When we slump the lumbar spine is forced out causing us to lose our natural lordosis. The result is a double imbalance of kyphosis and flatback.

Kyphosis and flatback don't always come together. A person can suffer with kyphosis but not sit all day, a nurse for example who is bending over regularly but also moving around could be subject to kyphosis from the bending but the other activities could cause a counter position in the spine causing lordosis. All these imbalances place excessive strain on the joints.

Problems
- Short/tight pecs (chest muscle)
- Lengthened trapezius muscle in the upper and middle fibers (causing round shoulders)
- Weak abdominals
- Weak gluteals (buttocks)
- Tension in neck and shoulders

Solution
- Stretch chest muscle
- Strengthen postural fibers in middle and lower trapezius
- Strengthen abdominals and gluteals (buttocks)
- Lengthen neck extensors, strengthen neck flexors

Exercises
- Standing heel raises
- Arm floats
- Standing twist
- Shoulder squeeze
- Shoulder roll down
- All fours
- Shell stretch
- Breast stroke prep
- Gluteal squeeze
- Side lying open door
- Skull rock
- Hamstring stretch
- Shoulder bridge
- Double arm circles
- Hip flexor stretch
- Monkey squat

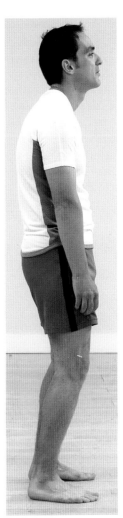

This posture shows a double imbalance of kyphosis and flatback.

15

SWAY BACK

The sway back posture is often known as the lazy posture. It is commonly adopted by teenagers and those who stoop because they are conscious of their height. It is also the posture that most catwalk models adopt which becomes an occupational posture.

The noticeable features of a sway back are sitting into the hip and favoring one leg when standing, allowing the abdominals to relax and lengthen. The head is usually held to one side rather than being central and the arms hang forward.

It gets the name lazy because those who have this posture can sometimes very easily correct it by standing tall and distributing their weight evenly through the legs. If the posture is long standing then there are considerable differences in the strength on one side of the body to the other. By favoring one leg, the muscles on one side will be shortening while on the other side they will be lengthening. The abdominal tone in sway backs is lax so all of the abdominal family will need conditioning to help correct this posture. It is the only posture where the hip flexors are likely to be lengthened and in need of strengthening, whereas in all the other postures the hip flexors need to be lengthened in order to release tension at the top of the legs.

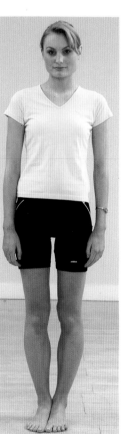
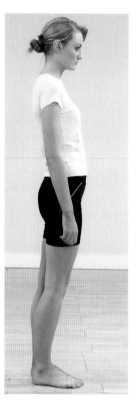

This posture shows the typical features of sway back from the front and side.

Problems
- Favors one leg when standing
- Lengthened hip flexors
- Tight hamstrings
- Lengthened abs/obliques
- Head slant

Solutions
- Strengthen all the abdominal group
- Strengthen the hip flexors
- Stretch the hamstrings
- Re-align neck position

Exercises
- Standing set position
- Heel raises
- Single leg balance
- Arm floats
- All fours: cat's tail
- Breast stroke prep
- Prone squeeze
- Shell stretch
- Side lying open door
- Skull rock
- Single leg stretch
- Obliques
- Hamstring stretch
- Shoulder bridge
- Shoulder squeeze
- Monkey squat

FLAT BACK

The flat back posture is just as it suggests—the back is flat, having lost the lordotic curve. It is seen in those who sit for prolonged periods especially if sitting in a slumped position, such as the coach potato or one who slumps in the office chair while making a telephone call. The muscles in the lumbar spine can become fixed quite quickly resulting in an inability to bend forward or backward freely. Due to this stiffness, mobility exercises need to be taken slowly and gently to encourage the spine to move and to regain its natural curve. When a flat back posture is identified, the pelvis is in a posterior tilt where the hip bones sit behind the level of the pubic bone causing the lumbar spine to lengthen. Those with flat back problems will complain that they cannot get up and move well after sitting or sleeping but are ok once they have been up for a while. The flat back posture very often accompanies the kyphotic posture, so you may have identified your own posture falling into these two groups.

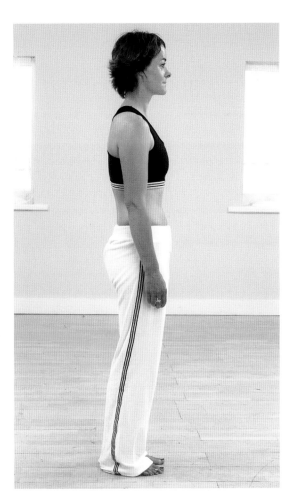

Problems
- Spine is fixed
- Lack of mobility, especially in extension
- Gluteal inhibition (weak buttocks)

Solutions
- Strengthen gluteals and abdominals
- Increase mobility and range of movement in area that is fixed
- Increase lordosis

Exercises
- Arm floats
- Standing heel raises
- Standing roll down from standing
- Seated "c" curve
- Hamstring stretch
- Shoulder bridge
- Hip roll
- Abdominal preparation
- Side lying open door
- Swimming legs and arms
- Breast stroke prep
- Swan dive
- All fours, cat's tail
- Shell stretch
- Monkey squat

The Five Basic Principles of Pilates

The five basic principles of Pilates educate you in how to hold the spine correctly during movement and will help to correct any imbalances that have been identified in your postural analysis.

These five principles are listed below:
1 Lateral (thoracic) breathing
2 Neutral pelvis
3 Rib cage placement
4 Scapula placement
5 Neck alignment

Lateral (Thoracic) Breathing

The power of breath

Breathing is one of our automatic functions that many take for granted and yet it is our primary source of energy. The way we breathe is mirrored in the way we live. Negative emotions can affect our breathing patterns and this has a knock on effect on our posture. You may have noticed when you are stressed or worried that your chest begins to tighten and your breath becomes shallow and faster increasing your heart rate. If we are calm the breathing and the heart rate is slower as we take the air deeper toward the abdomen using the diaphragm. Focusing on your breathing helps to increase the oxygen flow and rids us of the carbon dioxide in the blood. It increases our lung capacity and circulation. If our breathing is impeded then the flow of oxygen slows down allowing toxins to build gathering bacteria and causing congestion. Joseph Pilates realized the powerful connection between the mind and body and though we accept that the Eastern disciplines of yoga and t'ai chi use this in their own practice and have done for thousands of years, it was quite profound for a westerner to address this at the beginning of the twentieth century for general exercise prescription. It is now becoming widely accepted that breathing exercises have profound results in improving our physiological and psychological well being.

When the breath is calm, your moves are smooth and the body is relaxed and free of tension.

Mastering lateral breathing

Lateral breathing in Pilates is probably the most difficult to master and you will hear people comment on this that they just can't get it right, but it is really quite easy if you allow your breath to become natural. Most of the moves follow the natural rhythm of the body so it becomes logical to breathe in if we want to extend the spine and to breathe out when the body wants to flex.

Take a deep breath in and see what your body does. You will lift up when you breathe in and when you breathe out you relax.

As the principles of Pilates are on core stability we are using the deep lower abdomen muscles which prevent the breath from traveling down into the stomach. We are also concentrating on shoulder stability, which prevents the breath from staying high in the chest. So if it can't go down and it can't stay up, where does it go? It has to go out, laterally using the expansion of the rib cage. Should that area of the body be a little stiff then it can take some time for the intercostals to regain their elasticity so don't despair if you find this part difficult to begin with, persevere and you will achieve results.

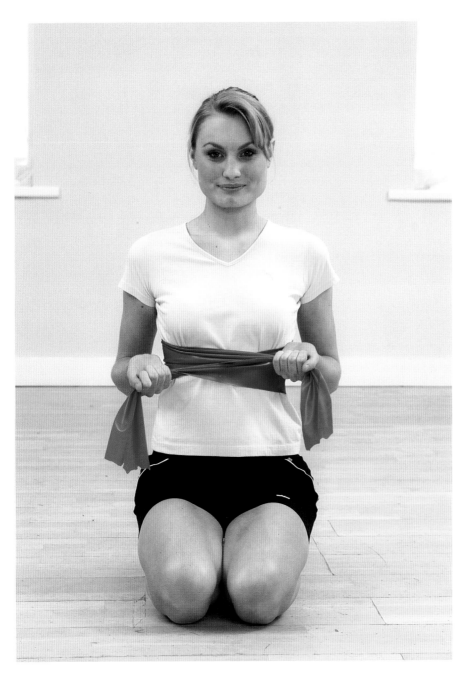

1 Place an exercise band or scarf around the rib cage as seen in the picture and cross it over in front. Have it wide across your back so you can feel it.

2 As you take a full breath in, take the breath into the band and feel it expand. The hands will come closer together as the band expands.

3 As you breathe
out pull the
band. You will
feel the ribs close
down and your
hands will go
further apart.

**Opening up the
ribs is essential for
full and healthy
breathing. Do this
in front of the
mirror and watch
your shoulders.
When you breathe
in don't allow the
shoulders to rise
up. Direct the
breath into the rib
cage and let them
expand like
bellows.**

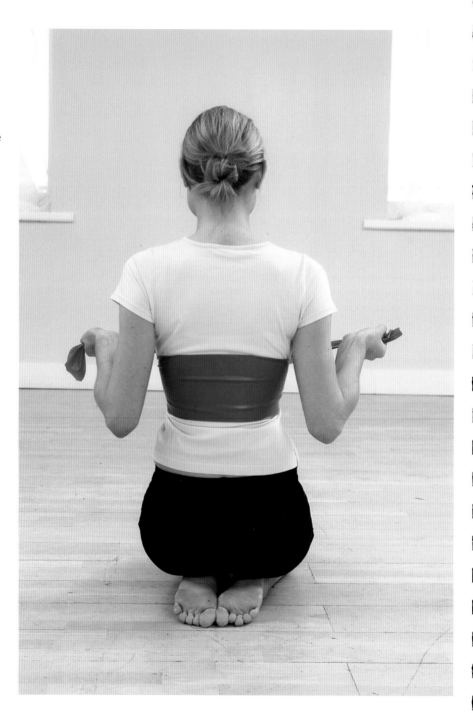

Neutral Pelvis

Assessing the alignment of your pelvis used to be down to the expertise of a doctor or a gynaecologist. We are now able to assess this ourselves. If you look at the diagram below it shows the neutral position where the hip bones, A.S.I.S. (anterior superior iliac spine) and the pubic bone are in a parallel line to one another. This means you will have a natural lordotic curve.

Posterior Tilt or Kyphotic Posture

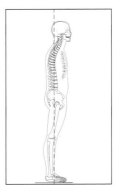

So in order to maintain a healthy back it is imperative that we try to restore neutral alignment.

Neutral Posture

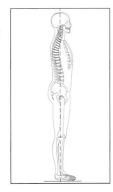

Finding a neutral pelvis

This can be done in a number of ways, but here are two ways to find a neutral pelvis.

If however the pelvis is in an anterior tilt (see below) and the hip bones are forward of the pubic bone, this will increase the lordotic curve of the spine, placing pressure on the lumbar discs.

Finding a neutral pelvis in a standing position

1   Stand with your feet parallel and hip width apart.
2   Keep your knees soft, not bent or locked out.
3   Keep your hands placed at the waist on top of the hip bones as if resting on top of a bucket of water.
4   Draw the shoulders down and keep the upper body still and stable.
5   Tilt the "bucket" to pour the water out of the front. You will feel your back arch creating an increase in the lordotic curve.
6   Now tilt the bucket back to pour the water out of the back so you now loosen the lordotic curve.
7   Continue with this a few times to feel the movement. You may be surprised at how small the move is when you don't allow the upper body to move. Shoulders stay still.
8   Bring the bucket to where you consider level. This will be your neutral pelvis.

Anterior Tilt or Lordotic Posture

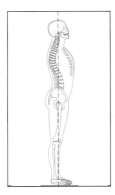

If the hip bones are sitting behind the pubic bone in a posterior tilt (see top right), the curve is lost and this puts strain on the lumbar discs.

Finding a neutral pelvis when lying down (supine)

1 Lie with your feet parallel.

2 Keep your knees bent in line with your hip bones.

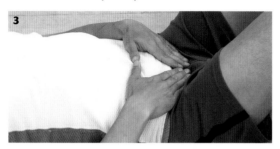

3 Place the heel of your hands on your hip bones, your fingers toward the pubic bone and thumbs toward the navel, forming the shape of a triangle.

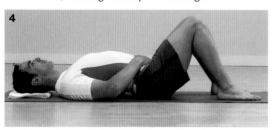

4 Place an imaginary marble into the triangle and roll it toward the fingers, arching the back.

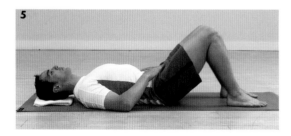

5 Now roll toward your thumbs and feel your back press into the mat. This is called imprinting.

6 Continue through those two ranges of movement.

7 Notice how much movement is going on in the upper body.

In Pilates we are aiming all the time to isolate the area we are working. If we have tight or weak muscles anywhere then the body is very clever at cheating. It will recruit other muscles to assist, so by making the movement less we are able to focus on that area and determine whether we are cheating or not. It's ok to cheat as long as you know you're doing it. Then you can start learning how not to.

So ask yourself during this exercise: "Can I roll the marble forward and back without moving my head or shoulders?" If the answer is "Yes," then you're not cheating. If the answer is "No," make the move smaller until the answer becomes "Yes."

You may be surprised at how little movement you have when not cheating.

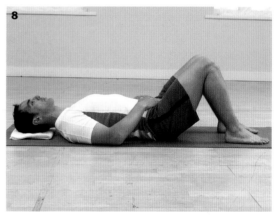

8 Bring your marble to the center of your triangle now. You should not be arching or imprinting. From the side, your hands should look level to the floor.

Rib Cage Placement

The ribs are ingeniously arranged to allow the movement required for breathing while also providing protection for the heart and lungs. When we breathe the ribs should move laterally like bellows which massages the internal organs. In fact with every breath the ribs should move freely in three ways, lifting, extending outward, and rotating along its axis. Unfortunately more often than not when we breathe the breath goes either down into the abdomen or it stays high in the chest raising the shoulders. If our ribs are stiff they will rise rather than expand causing the spine to extend. This in turn causes the pelvis to anteriorly tilt placing pressure on the lumbar discs. Correct placement of the rib cage is an essential contribution to the stability of the spine and therefore is a major player when it comes to correct alignment.

Rib cage placement while standing

1   Stand with your feet hip width apart.

2   Keep your knees soft and in line with your hip bones.

3   Your pelvis is in neutral.

4   Place your thumbs on your bottom rib.

5   Place your middle finger on your hip bone.

6   Draw your thumbs and ribs down toward your hips and fingers. (Your body will bend or flex forward.)

7   Open the distance between your thumbs and fingers. (Your body will extend and the back arch.)

8   Feel the movement coming from the rib cage.

9   Now stand upright and find a neutral pelvis. Find the gap between your ribs and hips and stay there for the correct rib cage placement.

If structurally your rib cage sits high, then you cannot change that but the fact your ribs sit high may be because you are slightly lordotic, as you are arching too much in your lower back. In this case as you work with these exercises, the back will start to re-align and the ribs will soften down.

Rib cage placement when lying down (supine)

1   Lie on your back with your knees bent.

2   Your feet are parallel in line with your knees and in line with the hips.

3   Keep your pelvis in neutral.

4   Place your hands on your ribs, your fingers touching.

5   Imagine your ribs are like butterfly wings. When you breathe in the wings open and when you breathe out the wings close.

6   If you find your bottom rib with your thumbs and your hip bones with your fingers, you will have a gap of about 4 inches (10cm).

7   Draw the ribs closer to the hips so the thumbs come closer to the fingers and your shoulders will want to lift off the floor. You are closing the gap and the body is beginning to flex.

8   If you expand the distance between your thumb and finger, the back will arch away from the floor and your ribs will flare.

9   Bring yourself back into a neutral pelvis position and just allow the ribs to soften down so the back is not over-arching nor imprinting.

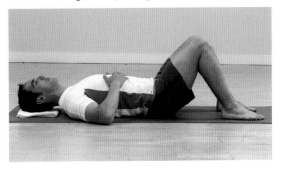

Scapula Placement

The shoulder blades (scapula) should ideally lie flat against the rib cage. They move quite freely upward/downward/outward/inward and rotate and the muscles that are attached to them are key players in shoulder stabilization.

If you look at the numerous muscles listed below that directly effect the position of the scapula, you will appreciate the complexity of diagnosis when a problem in the shoulder occurs.

Mid Fibers of Trapezius adduct and slightly elevate the scapula. Rhomboids also adduct the scapula. The Levator Scapulae works with the Trapezius to elevate and adduct. Serratus Anterior draws the scapula forward to sit against the ribs. The Deltoids abducts the shoulder and is attached to the spine of the scapula.

The Supraspinatus is attached to the spine too which helps the Deltoid in abducting the arm, also attached to the spine of the scapula. Teres Major adducts and medially rotates the Humerus. It is attached to the bottom edge of the scapula. Subscapularis originates inside the surface of the scapula. Teres Minor originates at the edge of the scapula and it laterally rotates the Humerus. Infraspinatus also laterally rotates the Humerus and it originates below the spine of the scapula.

In the event of any of these muscles becoming tight, short, or lengthened the scapula will be displaced.

Aligning the scapula

1 Stand in front of a mirror, feet hip width apart.
2 Keep your knees soft in line with your hip bones.
3 Keep your pelvis in neutral.
4 Keep your arms by your side.
5 Shrug the shoulders up to the ears.
6 Draw shoulders down and away from the ears.
7 Repeat a couple of times to focus on the shoulder blades rather than the shoulders. Feel them move up in your back when you shrug and move down when you release.

8 Visualize the scapula moving down your back.

Look in the mirror and see where the arms are. Press the middle finger into your leg gently. Now draw the shoulder blades together as tightly as possible and you will notice your fingers will shift around the leg. This shows you that the position and movement of the scapula affects the position of the arms.

Draw the shoulder blades toward one another again but only slightly and release. Keeping your shoulder blades moving down your back helps with shoulder stability and corrects faulty movement patterns in the upper body.

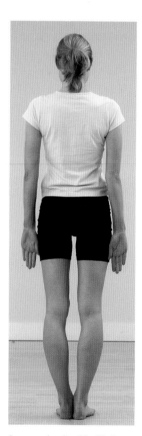
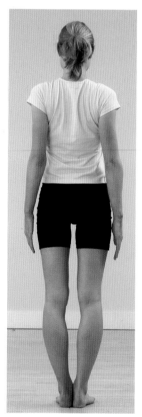

Squeeze the shoulder blades together.

Neck Alignment

The position of the head on top of the spine is extremely important. When correct the natural lordotic curve in the neck is present. The head weighs approximately 10–15lb (5kg), so if it is not centrally placed, the distribution through the first few vertebrae is doubled, sometimes tripled, causing overload and tension.

Ideally the head should sit centrally on top of the atlas, the first vertebrae, so the load can be evenly distributed down the spine.

Aligning the neck

1 Lie on your back with your knees bent.

2 Keep your feet in line with your knees and your knees in line with your hip bones.

3 Your pelvis is in neutral.

4 Your rib cage and scapula should be in correct alignment.

5 With your head resting on floor nod your chin toward your chest to create a double chin.

6 Slide your head back to look behind you.

7 Go through these two ranges of movement and stop where you feel the center is. Are you looking directly at the ceiling, or can you see more ceiling in front than behind or vice versa?

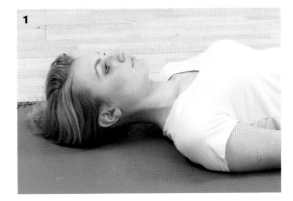

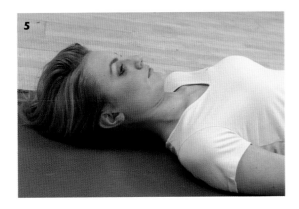

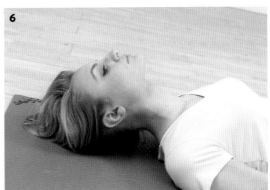

Aligning the neck (continued)

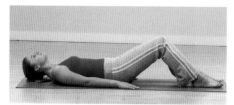

Head too far back.

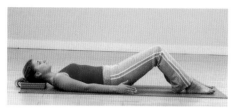

Head too high.

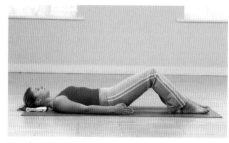

Head in alignment.

8 Use a towel or block under the head if you are looking at more ceiling behind than in front.

9 Think of holding a small peach under the chin to keep the alignment.

10 These learning procedures in alignment are exercises in their own right, so take your time to learn them.

Change is Strange

When we start to change the body's alignment it will feel strange, especially when learning the alignment exercises. The following exercise will demonstrate this:

1 Fold your arms.

2 Unfold them.

3 Now fold them again the other way.

How does it feel? Strange? Try this:

1 Clasp your hands together interlacing the fingers.

Which thumb is on top?

1 Clasp your hands together and place the other thumb on top.

Feel strange? That's because the first position was habitual; it was a movement so familiar that you did it without thinking. When we come to try and change these patterns it will feel strange and awkward to begin with because they are non habitual. To create a new movement pattern you have to do it three to five thousand times before the brain accepts it and it becomes automatic.

Learning the changes takes time. Pilates is not a quick fix to a new body. It is a lifestyle which means you have to give it time just as you did when you learnt to walk, to read, and to drive.

Abdominal Muscles and Core Stability

Our abdominal muscles are made up of four groups. The Rectus Abdominus, the External Obliques, the Internal Obliques, and the Transverse Abdominus (TA). Out of those muscles, the ones we focus on in Pilates are the deep stabilizing muscles, which are the Transverse Abdominus and Internal Obliques. The Rectus Abdominus and External Obliques form the superficial muscles which sit on top.

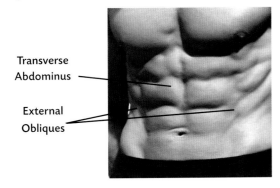

Transverse Abdominus

External Obliques

The Rectus Abdominus when defined gives the appearance of a "six pack" and the External Obliques allow us to twist and turn. Although these two superficial muscles are engaged when we perform any abdominal activity, the emphasis is concentrated on strengthening the Transverse Abdominus and the Internal Obliques. These two muscles form part of our internal corset along with the Multifidus muscles which sit close to the spine and our pelvic floor muscles, which are at the base of the torso and are explained in more detail a little further on.

The Transverse Abdominus when engaged attracts fibers from the Multifidus, Internal Obliques, and pelvic floor to create an internal girdle, along with the movement of the diaphragm. These muscles when working optimally create a cylinder inside the body holding the organs and spine in place. This is known as abdominal hollowing. If these muscles are not engaged during certain movements then the abdominals will dome in a sit up and if the pelvic floor is not drawn up, we will bear down causing flatulence. To learn how to do abdominal hollowing follow the exercises listed below. This can take time to master so look at doing this on a daily basis to begin with before starting your program.

Abdominal hollowing (standing)

1 Stand with your feet hip width apart.

2 Keep your knees in line with the hip bones.

3 Your rib cage is down.

4 Your shoulder blades are moving down your back.

5 Your neck is lengthened.

6 Take hold of the waist band of your shorts and pull them out in front of you.

7 Pull your abdominals in as tightly as you can, creating a big gap between yourself and your shorts. If you are pulling in as tightly as possible then it will be at 100 percent.

8 You will not be able to sustain this for very long so let it go.

9 Now pull in about 50 percent. You are now in a position to pull in to 100 percent if required. Let it go.

10 Now pull in at 25 percent. You know the muscle is switched on. You also know you could pull it in to 50 or 100 percent if needed. Let it go.

11 Now pull in again to 25 percent and continue breathing normally. Check every time you breathe out that you still have 25 percent engaged.

Initially try to do this up to 5 breaths until it becomes easier. Try this when standing, sitting, lying on your front, and on your back as you will be asked to do this when you come to learn the exercises. This is referred to throughout the book as tensing the Transverse Abdominis.

The Pelvic Floor Muscles

We all have pelvic floor muscles. They are attached to the inside of the pelvis and form a sling between the legs supporting our internal organs. If they were not there all our insides would fall out. The strength of these muscles are reduced in pregnancy and in very obese individuals. The tone of the muscle also reduces as we get older and gravity begins to take over, causing our internal organs to drop and rest on the muscles causing them to weaken. When the muscle is weak we experience incontinence when coughing, sneezing, or jumping. It is therefore important to regain control of the pelvic floor muscle and there is no age limit when this can be started. In Pilates we focus on this muscle while re-educating the other core stability muscles which form the internal corset.

Pelvic floor exercises

Learning how to use the pelvic floor again is an exercise in itself and should be performed as often as possible. Due to the fact it is an internal exercise, there should be no visible sign of you using it. To check the strength of your pelvic floor, next time you go to the bathroom, try and stop the flow of urine half way. The muscle you use to do this is the pelvic floor muscle. If you find this impossible you should consult your doctor to check the severity of the weakness, as it can lead toward prolapse and incontinence in both men and women and can be corrected quickly if acted upon. Try this exercise:

1 Lie on your back with your knees bent.
2 Relax the buttocks and the leg muscles.
3 Begin to tighten the muscle around the back passage as if you wanted to prevent flatulence.
4 Don't squeeze the buttocks when doing this.
5 Try to take this feeling now toward the front, the muscle you rely on when you need to prevent passing urine and there is no bathroom for miles.
6 Try to hold this for a couple of breaths and then relax.

Once you are familiar with these muscles you need to use them on a regular basis during the day. When sitting in the car, on your way to work, standing at the line in the supermarket, or just while you watch TV. Anywhere, anytime as it is extremely important to our health and well being.

The pelvic elevator

Think of the pelvic floor muscle as an elevator inside the body. When you engage the muscle the elevator comes up to the first floor. Hold it for at least one breath before relaxing back to the ground floor. As it gets stronger it will feel as if it is coming up to the second floor. Try not to let it drop back down, release it slowly.

Importance of working the pelvic floor

The exercise above helps us to work the pelvic floor slowly and with control—by doing this we are increasing the fibers known as slow twitch. These fibers increase the stamina within the muscle and help to sustain its strength. As we get older we are fighting against gravity and our internal organs are not exempt, they rely on the pelvic floor and core stabilizers to keep them in place. If the muscle weakens the organs begin to drop and in severe cases cause prolapse and incontinence. The exercise above helps to strengthen the slow twitch fibers and assists in core strength.

We also have fast twitch fibers which we rely on in cases of emergency. For example, when we cough, sneeze, slip, or jump, the fast twitch fibres switch on to prevent us from passing urine or wind involuntarily. Therefore they too need conditioning. To increase our fast twitch fibers we do the same kind of exercise as the pelvic elevator but quickly. Like a light switch, switching on, off, on, off. You pull up, release, pull up, release. Both these exercises can be done anywhere at any time.

The Ten Commandments of Set-up Positions

When starting any of the exercises you need to be in correct alignment. It is pointless executing an exercise if the body is incorrectly placed. You need to go through the ten commandments listed below before you start an exercise in a new position. You will also find these instructions within the routines listed in the next section. This will become very automatic in time but it is important to follow the ten commandments every time you change position.

1 Keep your feet apart in line with your knees.
2 Keep your knees in line with your hip bones.
3 Your pelvis should be in its neutral position.
4 Engage the Transverse Abdominus.
5 Your rib cage is soft and down.
6 Keep your shoulders away from your ears, arms by your side. (When on "all fours" keep your hands directly under your shoulders and when on your side keep your arms at shoulder level.)
7 Your shoulder blades are down.
8 Keep your chin in and neck long.
9 Breathe in to prepare. Breathe out to move.
10 Your pelvic floor is engaged.

All these positions follow the ten commandments. These are your set positions before starting an exercise.

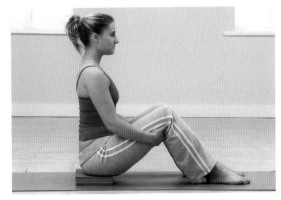

You can sit on a block with your knees bent to make sure the spine is neutrally aligned.

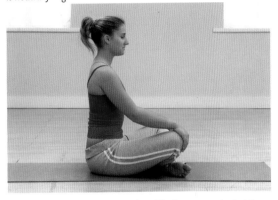

Alternatively you can cross your legs. The importance is that the spine is in its neutral position.

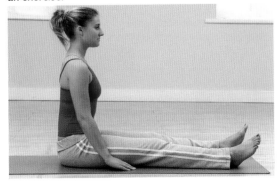

This is the full, seated set position.

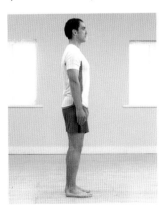

Standing set position.

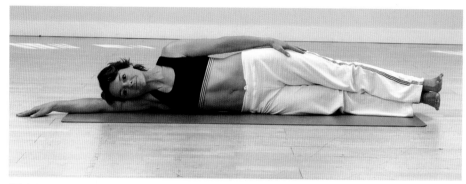

Side lying set 1 position.

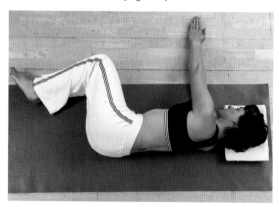

Side lying set 2 position.

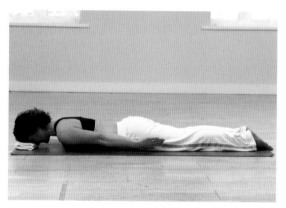

Prone set position.

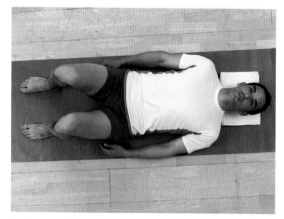

Supine set position.

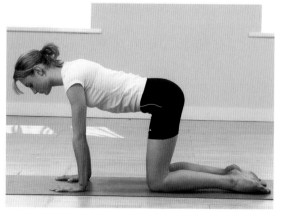

All fours set position.

Some Alternatives to Help You Get in Line

Depending on your posture type, there may be times when you will require either a towel or maybe a block under the head in order for it to be in correct alignment.

Similarly you may need a towel under the hips or feet to make the position more comfortable and to get you into a good alignment.

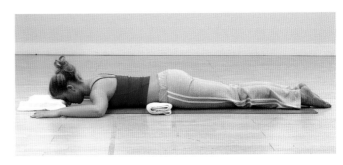

When lying on your front, the lower back can be put into an over lordotic position and can cause pinching.

Placing a rolled up towel under the hips can eliminate this problem as it helps to lengthen the lumbar spine.

If you have a knee problem, a towel can make this position more comfortable.

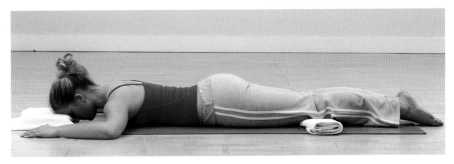

If you have inflexibility in the ankles, a towel under the foot had be of great benefit and comfort.

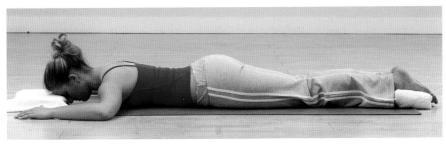

When lying on your front it is important to have something under your head to keep the neck and head in its correct alignment to the shoulders.

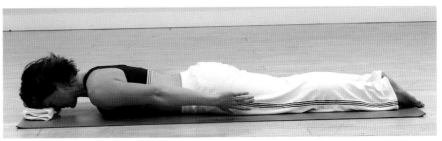

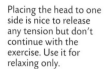

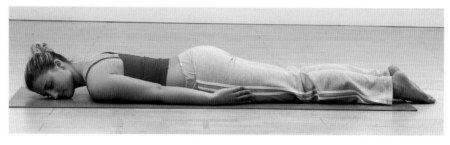

Placing the head to one side is nice to release any tension but don't continue with the exercise. Use it for relaxing only.

The towel under the head shows the neck in good alignment.

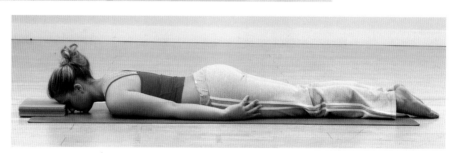

Whereas the block under the head shows the head sitting too high and the neck is shortened which will cause tension.

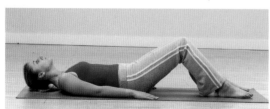

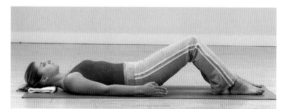

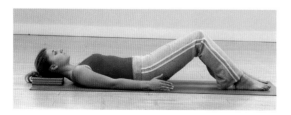

These three pictures show alignment in the neck when lying supine. One shows the neck tilted back which indicates that something is required under the head to lengthen the neck. The picture showing the block under the head shows that this correction is too high. Whereas the picture with the towel under the head shows good alignment.

Sitting upright without tension can prove extremely difficult for most people. This will be due to a number of factors.

• Poor abdominal tone
• Weak back muscles
• Tight hamstrings and hip flexors
• Kyphotic posture

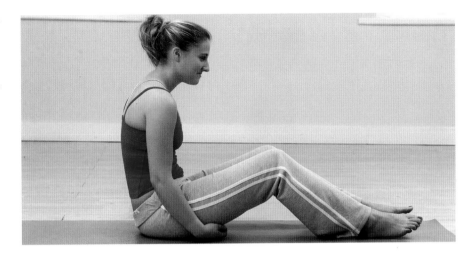

Using a block or even sitting on a chair if necessary will help to bring the back into a better position. Use a chair if needed for any of the sitting exercises or, better still, use a stability ball.

When sitting either have the legs crossed or bent out in front where you can place the hands under the thighs to help lift you up.

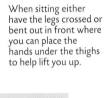

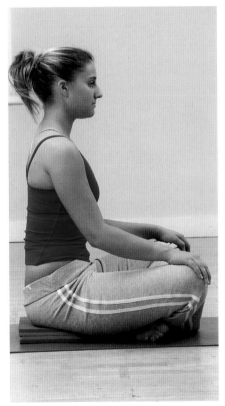

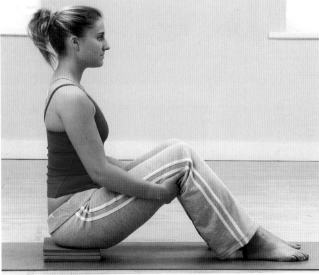

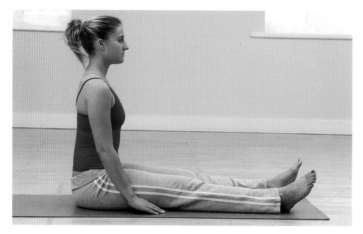

This is the autonomous sitting position.

Stretching in the shell stretch is great if you have no problems with your knees or hips. If you have difficulty in doing the shell stretch opt for hugging your knees into your chest.

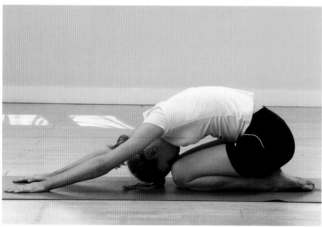

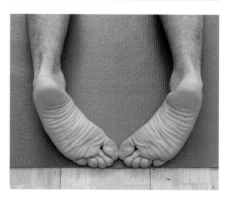

The prone squeeze. Asks for heels together then heels apart. This is part of the exercise but when you're not using the legs choose either parallel or pigeon toes for comfort.

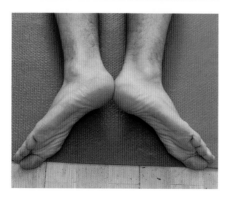

Before You Start

You need to know before starting a new program if it is suitable for you. If you have any concerns regarding your medical condition, you need to consult your doctor and ask advice. Although Pilates is ideal for those with conditions as mentioned earlier, it is just like any other exercise program where there is a level of risk involved and certain conditions need extra care and attention.

If you follow the guidelines and you are careful with the progressions then you will see great results.

Take time to pre-read the basic principles and try them one by one initially as they are exercises in their own right. The exercises themselves won't work as effectively if the five basic principles are not in place.

Try to pick a time when you know you will not be disturbed. Maybe turn off your cell phone so you have no distractions. Ideally we want to work and learn in a peaceful environment where you can concentrate on what you're doing and more importantly what you're feeling. Pilates is an integration of mind and body and the more relaxed we can be the better the benefits will be.

Equipment Needed

You don't need a lot of equipment but having some basic essentials will make things easier for you.

Firstly, you need enough space to be able to lie on your back and have room to outstretch your legs. You also need room to extend your arms over your head comfortably and out to the side without having any obstacles in your way.

- A large bath towel or exercise mat to lie on. If using a towel fold it over so you have some cushioning to support the whole back.
- A small towel to use under the head when needed.
- A long scarf or exercise band.

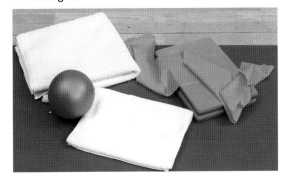

- A small soft ball or cushion.
- A yoga block or telephone directory to sit on.
- Some peace and quiet. Take the phone off the hook and turn your cell phone to silent.
- Wear something comfortable so as not to restrict your movements as any tight clothing will be uncomfortable.
- It is nice to have some background music playing. Choose something relaxing and avoid having any music with vocals or a hard beat. Quiet music playing does help relax both the mind and the body.

Put aside a place for your equipment so it is handy each time you come to practice. If you put stuff away it is a great excuse not to do your routine but if its out it reminds you. There are a variety of exercises and a number of ways to perform them. All the exercises shown are at a beginners level. Some of the exercises are preparation exercises for others that require a little more skill. You should learn the beginners exercises first before attempting the intermediate ones. Even then use them with discretion according to your condition.

30-Minute Routine For Lordotic Posture Types

These exercises are excellent for those who are on their feet for prolonged periods of time. It is also beneficial for people who do gymnastics, dancing, or running.

This routine is as follows:

- Supine set position
- Pelvic tilt
- Knee drop
- Hamstring stretch
- Shoulder bridge
- Ab prep
- Seated "c" curve
- Seated spine twist
- Roll down/ roll up
- Cat pedals
- Shell stretch
- Cat's tail
- Hip flexor stretch
- Hip flexor stretch 2
- Arm floats
- Monkey squat

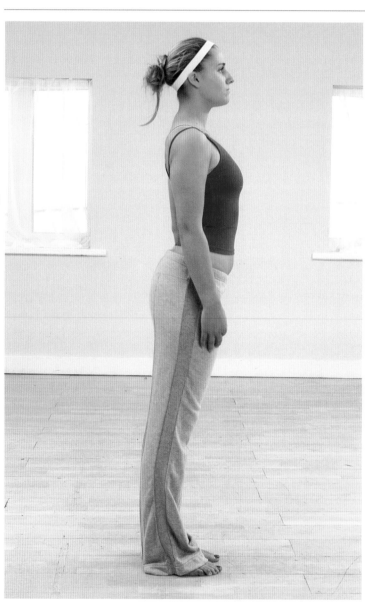

supine set position
Beginner

Objective: To establish good alignment of the spine and to practice the Ten Commandments of Pilates.

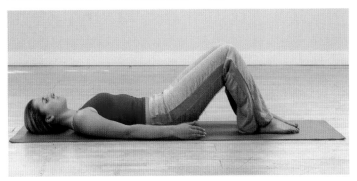

Start Position

- Supine set position.
- Feet apart in line with your knees.
- Knees in line with your hip bones.
- Pelvis in its neutral position.
- Transverse Abdominus is slightly tensed (or engaged).
- Rib cage soft and down.
- Shoulders away from the ears, arms by your side.
- Shoulder blades down and slightly tensed (engaged).
- Chin down, neck long.
- Breathe in and breathe out.
- Pelvic floor slightly tensed.

Technique

1 Breathe in.
2 Breathe out to contract abdominals and draw up the pelvic floor.
3 Breathe in.
4 Breathe out to relax.

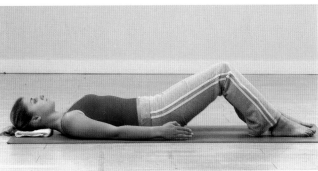

Alternative start position: Use a towel if needed.

Repetitions

- Initially 10 times, reducing as it becomes more automatic.

Hints & Tips
- Take your time to feel muscles tensing.

37

pelvic tilt
Beginner

Objective: To increase mobility in the lumbar spine and to strengthen the core stability muscles.

Start Position

- Supine set position.

Technique

1 Breathe in keeping pelvis neutral.
2 Breathe out and tense (engage) Transverse Abdominus and pelvic floor. Tilt the pelvis to imprint the spine.
3 Breathe in.
4 Breathe out to return to neutral pelvis and relax.

Repetitions

- Repeat 10 times, reducing to 5 as it becomes automatic.

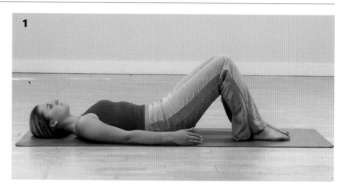

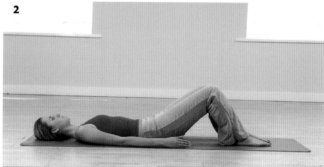

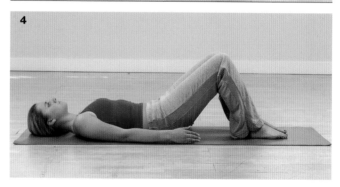

Hints & Tips
- Keep neck alignment by maintaining the gap between chin and chest.
- Don't squeeze the buttocks.

knee drop
Beginner

Objective: To strengthen core stabilizers by moving legs and to mobilize the hip.

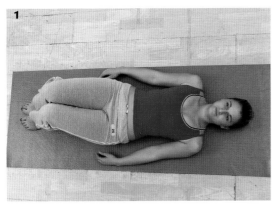

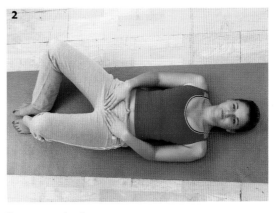

Start Position

- Supine position with feet together.
- Knees pointing straight up.

Technique

1 Breathe in.
2 Breathe out to engage Transverse Abdominus and pelvic floor. Drop the right knee slowly out to the side.
3 Breathe in and hold position.
4 Breathe out, moving knee back up and relax.
5 Repeat with other leg.

Repetitions

- 5 times with each leg.

Hints & Tips

- Hips stay still and stable.
- Supporting leg stays still and does not drop out at the same time as the moving leg. Imagine carrying a glass on the supporting knee while moving the other leg.
- Place hands on the hip bones to detect movement or place in the triangle position to help keep hips still.

hamstring stretch
Beginner

Objective: To lengthen the hamstring and to develop core strength and trunk stability.

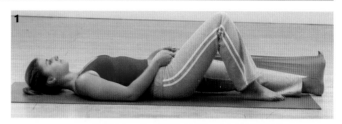

Start Position

- Supine position with one leg extended. Place an exercise band or long scarf around the extended leg.

Technique

1 Breathe in to prepare.

2 Breathe out to tense Transverse Abdominus and pelvic floor. Raise the leg slowly off the floor maintaining neutral alignment in the spine.

3 Continue to lift the leg toward a 90-degree angle, but only lift as high as comfortable, without raising the bottom or tilting the pelvis.

4 Breathe in for 3–5 breaths.

5 Breathe out and tense Transverse Abdominus and pelvic floor. Return leg to the floor and relax.

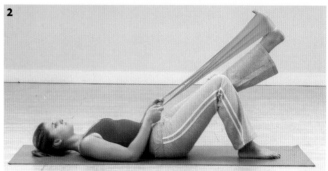

Repetitions

- 3–5 times on each leg.

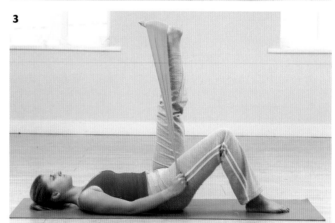

Hints & Tips

- Keep the pelvis in its neutral position.
- Keep the buttocks on the floor.
- Shoulders relaxed.
- Chin tucked slightly to keep length in the back of the neck.

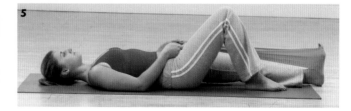

shoulder bridge
Intermediate

Objectives: Segmental control of the spine to increase mobility. To develop core strength and strengthen the gluteals (buttocks) and hamstrings. To strengthen trunk stability and lengthen the hip flexors.

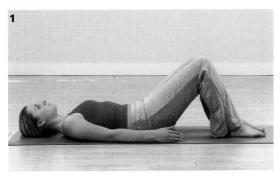

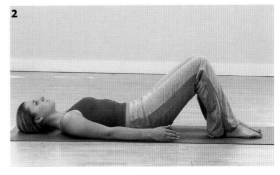

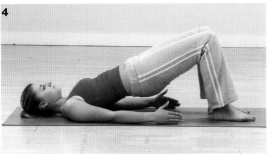

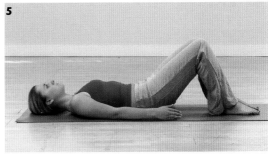

Start Position

- Supine set position. If you are using a block under the head for neck alignment, take it away for this exercise. If you are using a folded towel, leave it where it is.

Technique

1 Breathe in to prepare.
2 Breathe out to tense the Transverse Abdominus and pelvic floor. Tilt the pelvis, as in the pelvic tilt, to imprint the spine.
3 Breathe in.
4 Breathe out and tense Transverse Abdominus and pelvic floor. Squeeze the buttocks and lift off the floor, peeling one vertebrae off at a time, lifting toward the shoulder blades.

5 Breathe in and then breathe out to tense Transverse Abdominus and pelvic floor. Move back to the floor sequentially, returning the spine to neutral.

Repetitions

- Start with 5 and increase to 10.

Hints & Tips

- It is a slow exercise so take as many breaths as you need but keep checking that the abdominals are hollowed and the pelvic floor tensed. As a rule, stop to take a breath in and continue on the out breath.
- Check the weight distribution between your feet to see if you are favoring one side at any time.
- Only ever go up as high as is comfortable.
- Don't allow the ribs to flare as you get higher off the floor.

abdominal preparation
Beginner

Objective: To strengthen the Transverse Abdominus by maintaining abdominal hollowing while lifting the head. Also strengthens the core and shoulder stabilizers and the deep neck flexors. This is a good preparation exercise for all moves that require you to lift the head and shoulders off the floor.

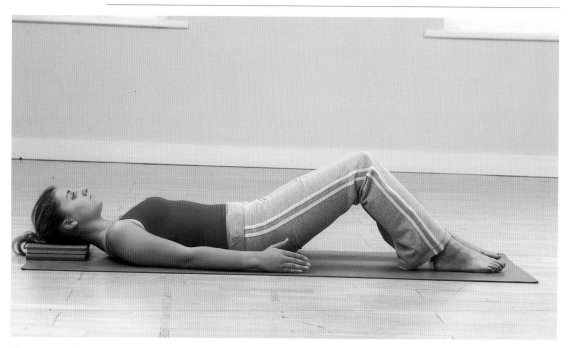

Start Position

- Supine set position.

Note:

Here, you are asked to lift your head off the floor which requires strength in the neck flexors to keep correct alignment. If you are using a towel under the head for correct neck placement before you start, you may find that by folding the towel so it sits higher under the head or by using a block it will keep the head in better alignment, especially on the return of the head to the floor.

This picture does show the head sitting too high, but for the abdominal prep exercise it will help in assisting correct placement of the neck on the return. This will help strengthen the neck flexors so eventually you won't need anything under the head at all.

Technique

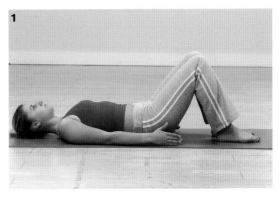

1 Breathe in to prepare.

2 Breathe out to engage Transverse Abdominus and pelvic floor.

3 Breathe in, drop chin slightly to chest.

4 Breathe out to slide the ribs toward the hips and hands toward the ankles, lifting the head and shoulders, looking toward the knees.

Modifications
• If you suffer with neck or shoulder problems do not lift the head off the floor. Continue with everything else—just omit the lifting of the head and shoulders.

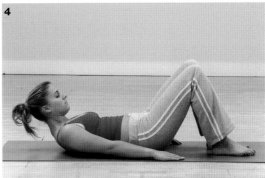

Hints & Tips

• Don't raise the head and shoulders if the abdominals are doming.
• Use the modification if you have any neck or shoulder problems.
• Buttocks stay relaxed.
• Pelvis stays in neutral.
• Don't forget the skull rock before lifting the head.

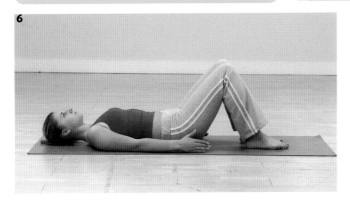

5 Breathe in to return.

6 Breathe out to release and relax.

Repetitions

• Start with 5 and build up to 10 as it can be very tiring on the neck muscles.

43

seated "c" curve
Beginner

Objectives: To strengthen the abdominals and develop core strength. Helps to mobilize and strengthen the spinal muscles and the shoulder stabilizers while sitting.

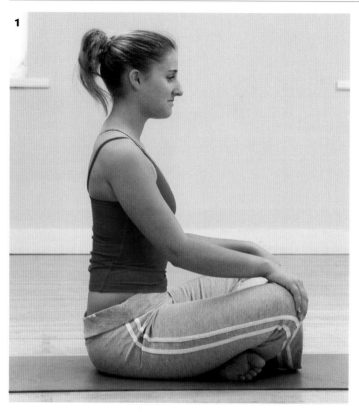

If you are slumping then use a block.

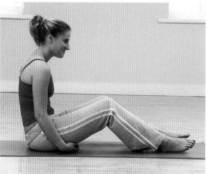

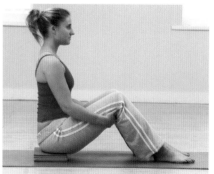

44

Start Position

- Seated set position.
- Legs crossed or knees bent and apart.
- Knees in line with your hip bones unless they are crossed.
- Pelvis in neutral position.
- Transverse Abdominus engaged.
- Rib cage soft and down.
- Shoulders away from the ears, hands resting on the knees.
- Shoulder blades down and slightly tensed.
- Chin down, neck long.
- Breathe in and out.
- Pelvic floor engaged.

Technique

1 Breathe in to prepare.
2 Breathe out to engage the Transverse Abdominus and pelvic floor, tilting the pelvis to create a "c" curve in the spine.
3 Breathe in to lift and return to neutral spine.

Repetitions

- Start with 5 and build up to 10 as this can be tiring on the hip flexors and spinal muscles.

Hints & Tips

- Initiate the movement from the pelvis not the shoulders.
- The shoulders stay over the hips during the movement, as seen in the picture (ask someone to check or watch yourself side on in the mirror). Keep an imaginary line from the shoulder to side of hip when sitting upright and when in "c" curve.

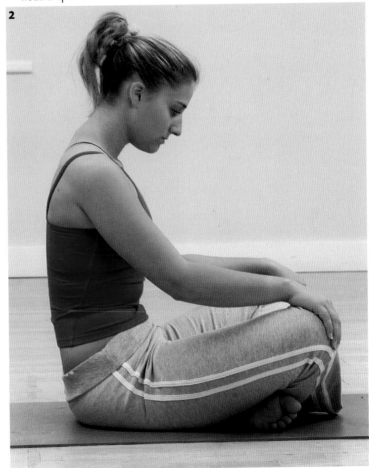

45

seated spine twist
Beginner

Objective: To mobilize the spine in rotation while maintaining stability and strength. It also strengthens trunk stability and develops core strength.

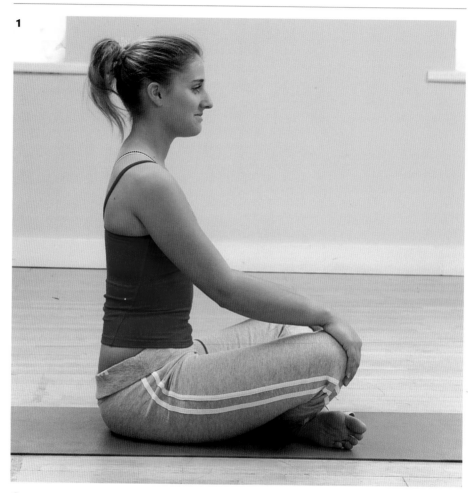

1

Start Position

- Seated set position—use towel or block if required to attain neutral spine.

2

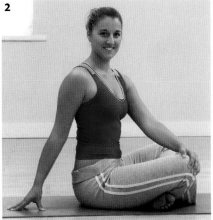

3

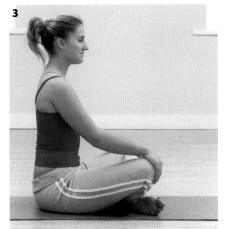

4

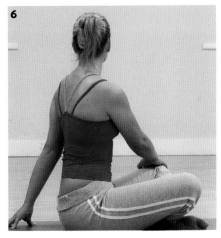

6

Technique

1 Breathe in
  to prepare.

2 Breathe out to
  engage Transverse
  Abdominus and
  pelvic floor. Twist
  from the waist
  slowly to the right,
  turning head to
  the right too.

3 Breathe in to
  return to center.

4 Add a "c" curve
  here if the hip
  flexors or back
  feel tired.

5 Breathing in,
  return to an
  upright position.

6 Breathe out and
  engage Transverse
  Abdominus and
  pelvic floor.
  Turn to your left.

7 Breathe in to
  return to center
  again (adding a
  "c" curve if needed
  for release).

Repetitions

• Start with a few to begin with and
  progress to 5 on each side.

Hints & Tips

• Very tiring in hip flexors and back muscles
  so include a "c" curve when at center to
  release.
• Don't lean back when rotating.
• Keep arms low to assist in shoulder
  stability.

47

roll down/roll up
Intermediate

Objectives: To strengthen abdominals and the spinal muscles during flexion and mobilize the spine segmentally. To strengthen all torso stabilizers and develop core strength.

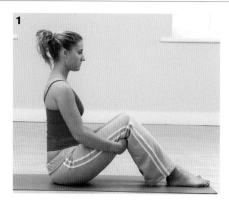

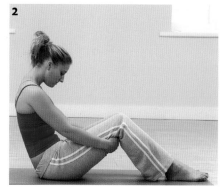

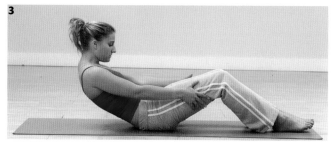

Start Position

• Seated set position with knees in front.

Technique

1 Breathe in to prepare.

2 Breathe out to engage Transverse Abdominus and pelvic floor. Tilt the pelvis to create a "c" curve.

3, 4, & 5 Continue to roll down segmentally toward the floor, keeping your feet down.

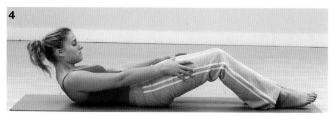

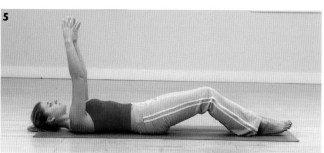

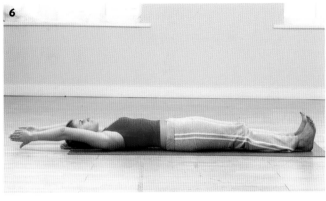

6 Breathe in to lengthen the legs away, taking the arms up and over the head, keeping the rib cage down.

7 Breathe in for skull rock and raise arms to the ceiling.

8 Slide the ribs toward the hip, lifting the head and shoulders and peeling the spine up off the floor one vertebrae at a time.

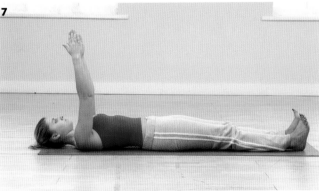

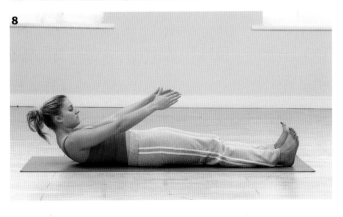

roll down/roll up (continued)

9 Tilt the pelvis on the way up to get good segmental control.

10 Breathe out as you roll up and stretch toward the toes, sliding the shoulder blades back away from the ears, head between the arms—bend the knees if needed.

11 Breathe in to start rolling back.

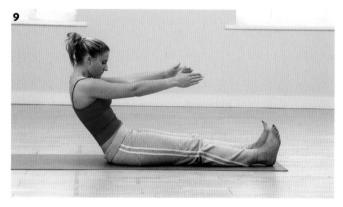

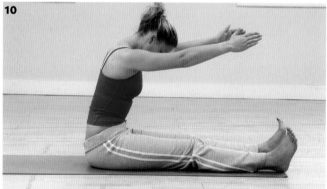

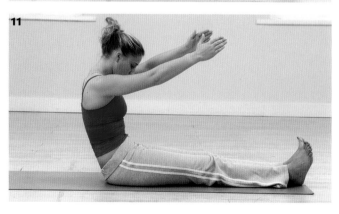

12

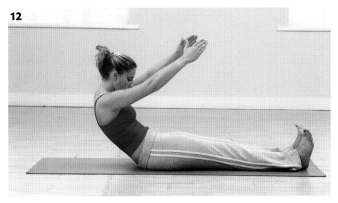

13

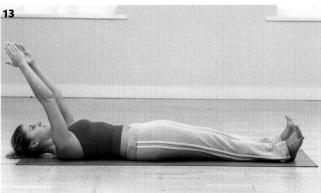

14

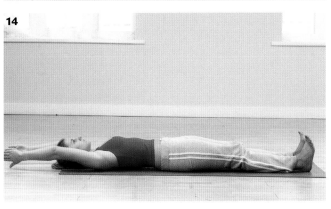

12, 13, & 14 Breathe out and tense Transverse Abdominus and pelvic floor as you roll back down toward the floor. Finishing with the arms back over the head, keeping the rib cage down.

Repetitions

- Do 10 repetitions. The "c" curve and the abdominal preparations are good practice for this exercise.

Hints & Tips

- Don't use momentum to get up off the floor, use control and strength.
- Maintain abdominal hollowing throughout the movement.

cat pedals
Beginner

Objectives: To strengthen all trunk stabilizers, focusing mainly on shoulder stability and develop core strength. To "bone load" (increase the density of the bones) the upper body, strengthen the spinal extensors, and develop balance and strength.

1

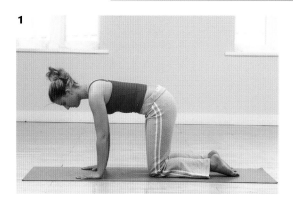

2

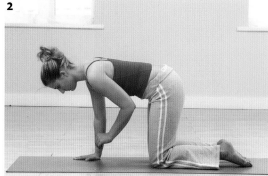

Start Position

- All fours set position.
- Feet apart in line with your knees.
- Knees in line with your hip bones.
- Pelvis in its neutral position.
- Transverse Abdominus slightly tensed.
- Rib cage soft and down.
- Shoulders away from the ears, hands directly under the shoulders.
- Chin down, neck long.
- Breathing in and out.
- Pelvic floor engaged.

Technique

1 Breathe in to prepare.
2 Breathe out to engage Transverse Abdominus and pelvic floor. Raise the left hand off the floor, bending at the elbow to avoid moving the shoulders.
3 Breathe in and replace the hand on the floor.
4 Breathe out, engage Transverse Abdominus and pelvic floor and raise the right hand.
5 Breathe in to replace the hand again.

3

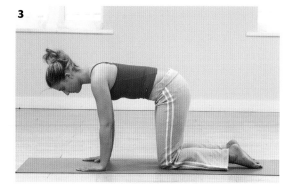

Repetitions

- Start with 5 on each hand and progress to 10 before taking a rest in the shell stretch. This can be very tiring on the wrists.

Hints & Tips

- Keep the spine still and stable while raising the hands.
- Don't take the weight back onto legs while raising the hands.
- There should be no visible movement anywhere other than the arms.

shell stretch
Beginner

Objectives: To stretch and release back extensors.

Technique

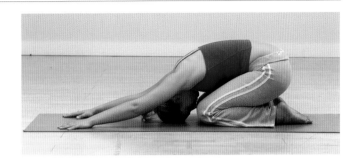

1 Breathe in and out while in this position, keeping the body relaxed.

Modifications
• If you have knee problems, roll onto your back or side and hug knees into chest.

cat's tail
Beginner

Objectives: To strengthen all trunk stabilizers, focusing mainly on shoulder stability and to develop core strength and bone load the upper body. It also strengthens the spinal extensors.

Technique

1 Get in all four set position.
2 Breathe in to prepare.
3 Breathe out to engage Transverse Abdominus and pelvic floor and tilt the pelvis, tucking the tail under, keeping the upper back stable and still.
4 Breathe in to bring the pelvis back into a neutral position.

Repetitions

• Start with 5 and progress toward 10 before taking a rest in shell stretch.

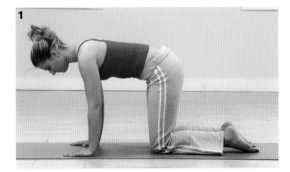

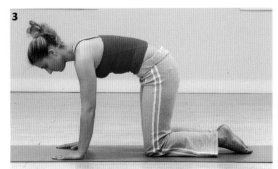

Hints & Tips
• Keep the upper body still and stable.
• Movement is small.
• Watch the lower back doesn't sag when coming back into neutral.

hip flexor stretch
Beginner

Objectives: To lengthen the hip flexor muscle

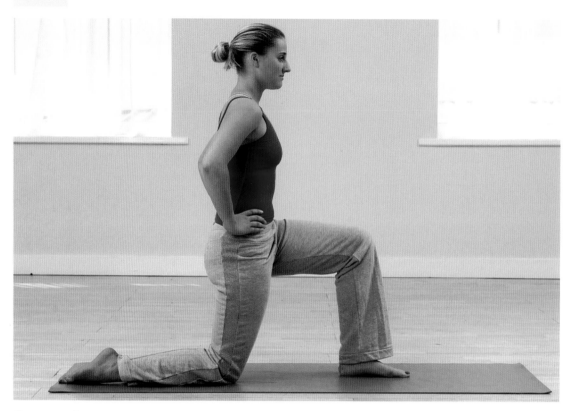

Start Position

• Kneeling with one leg in front.

Repetitions

• 3 times on each leg.

Technique

1 With one leg in front, knee bent at a 90-degree angle and in line with the ankle.

2 Breathe in with pelvis and spine neutral.

3 Engage abdominals and pelvic floor.

4 Tuck tail bone under until you feel mild tension at the front of the leg.

5 Hold stretch for 2–3 breaths and release.

Hints & Tips

• Keep angle in front leg so knee does not go over the toes.
• Weight is equally distributed between the legs.
• Place the supporting knee slightly back to increase stretch.

hip flexor stretch 2
Beginner

Objectives: Provides an alternative position for the hip flexor stretch if you are unable to kneel on the floor.

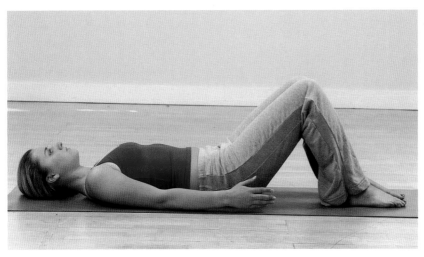

Start Position

• Supine set position.

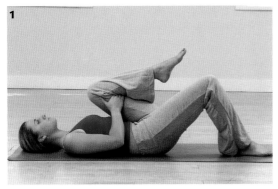

1

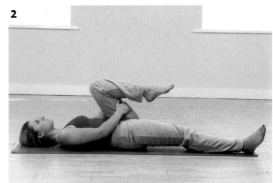

2

Technique

1 Breathe in and bring one knee up toward the chest.
2 Breathe out to lengthen the other leg away along the floor, keeping the other knee close to the chest.
3 Hold for 2–3 breaths and repeat on the other side.

55

arm floats
Beginner

Objectives: To strengthen shoulder stability and mobilize the shoulder joint.

Start Position

- Start in the standing set position.
- Your feet are apart in line with your knees.
- Your knees are in line with your hip bones.
- Your pelvis is in a neutral position.
- Engage the Transverse Abdominus muscles.
- Your rib cage is soft and down.
- Keep your shoulders away from your ears, arms by your side.
- Keep your shoulder blades down and engaged.
- Tuck your chin in to keep your neck long.
- Breathe in to prepare and breathe out to move.
- Engage your pelvic floor.

Technique

1 Breathe in.
2 Breathe out and engage the Transverse Abdominus and pelvic floor muscles and raise your arms to shoulder height
3 Breathe in to lower the arms back down to your side.

Repetitions

- 5–10 times.

Hints & Tips

- Your shoulders stay down while lifting the arms.
- Your weight stays equally distributed between your feet.
- Your rib cage stays down.
- Your thumbs lead the way. Imagine helium balloons lifting the arms so they float up.

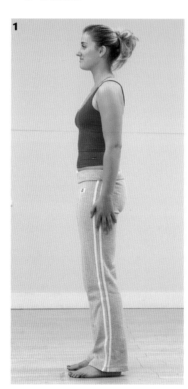

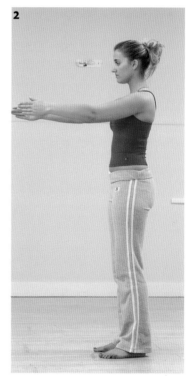

monkey squat
Beginner

Objectives: To develop good lifting skills, strengthening the trunk stabilizers while bending.

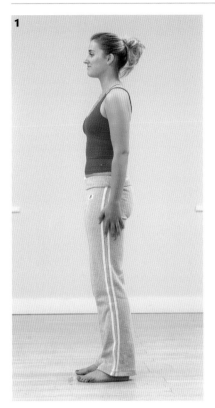

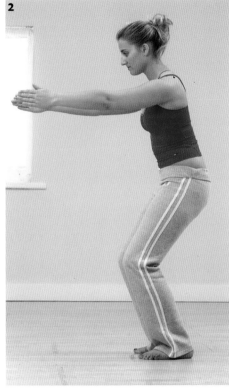

Modifications
- Keep your arms down so they follow the seam of the trousers as you bend.
- Take your arms behind your back to assist in keeping the shoulders back.

Start Position

- Stand in the standing set position.

Technique

1 Breathe in.
2 Breathe out and engage the Transverse Abdominus and pelvic floor muscles and hinge from the hip, taking the bottom back and bending the knees. The arms lift to shoulder level, leading with the thumbs.
3 Breathe in to return to standing.

Repetitions

- Start with 5 and progress to 10.

Hints & Tips
- The spine stays neutral.
- Bend at the knees, not the waist.
- Keep the shoulders in line with hips.

57

30-Minute Routine For Kyphotic Posture Types

These exercises focus on people who sit for prolonged periods during the day, for example office workers and drivers.

This routine is as follows:

- Standing heel raises
- Foot pedals
- Arm floats
- Standing twist
- Shoulder squeeze
- Half roll down
- Full roll down
- Cat pedals
- Side pocket
- Shake hands
- Toe pointing
- All fours balance
- Shell stretch
- Breast stroke preparation
- Prone squeeze
- Side lying open door
- Skull rock
- Hamstring stretch
- Double arm circles
- Shoulder bridge
- Hip flexor stretch
- Monkey squat

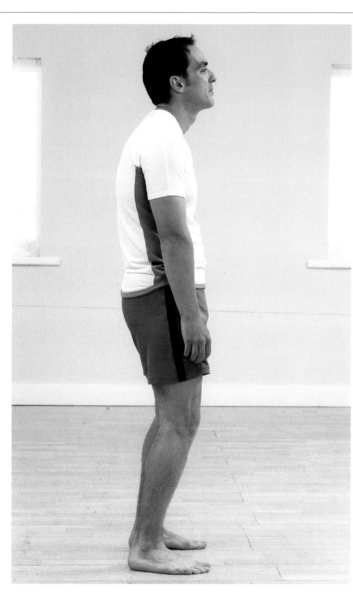

standing heel raises
Beginner

Objectives: To strengthen the Gluteus Medius muscle and to help prevent the pelvis from shifting involuntarily when walking or climbing stairs. To strengthen and mobilize the ankles and to strengthen the core stabilizers.

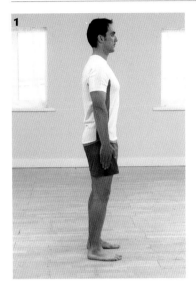
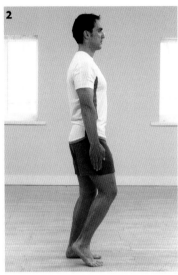
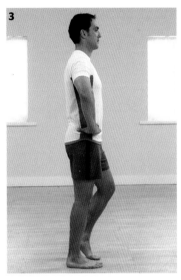

Start Position

- Stand with your feet apart in line with your knees in the standing set position.
- Your knees are in line with your hip bones.
- Your pelvis is in its neutral position.
- Engage the Transverse Abdominus muscles.
- Keep your rib cage soft and down.
- Keep your shoulders away from your ears, arms by your side.
- Your shoulder blades are down.
- Tuck your chin in and keep your neck long.
- Breathe in and breathe out.
- Engage the pelvic floor muscles.

Technique

1. Breathe in to prepare.
2. Breathe out and engage the Transverse Abdominus and pelvic floor muscles. Raise one heel

Hints & Tips

- Don't shift your weight from one hip to the other.
- Keep your weight distribution even through the legs. When you lift the heel, the weight should just transfer into the ball of the foot.
- It can get tiring on the ankles. The feet are always supported in shoes and the muscles rely on that support. When we come to work without support, the ankles fatigue quickly.

away from the floor. Breathe in to place the heel down.

3. Breathe out and engage the Transverse Abdominus and pelvic floor muscles to raise the other heel. Placing the hands on the hip bones gives you some awareness of any movement that is happening in the pelvis while changing from leg to the other. Your aim is to feel no movement in the pelvis at all.
4. Breathe in replace the foot.
5. Breathe out to engage the Transverse Abdominus and pelvic floor muscles, while you raise the other heel.

Repetitions

- 5–10 times.

foot pedals
Intermediate

Objectives: To strengthen the ankles and develop mobility, strengthen the stability of the hips, and increase the strength of the Gluteal Medius muscle which helps to stabilize the pelvis.

Start Position

- Start in the standing set position.

Technique

1 Breathe in to prepare.
2 Breathe out to engage the Transverse Abdominus and pelvic floor and raise the right heel off the floor.
3 Breathe in to engage the Transverse Abdominus and pelvic floor and raise the left heel to balance.
4 Breathe out to lower the right foot and bend the left knee, keeping the left heel up. Again this can be done with the arms by your side or for awareness keep the hands resting on the hip bones.

Repetitions

- 5–10 times depending on the strength of the ankles

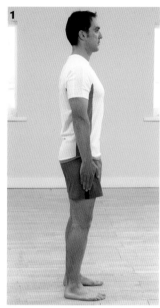
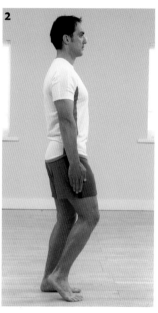
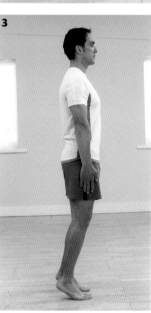
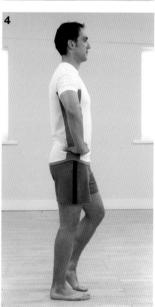

Hints & Tips

- Try to move straight up and straight down rather than shifting from side to side.
- Imagine you are between two planes of glass and you can only go up and down.
- When the hands are resting on the hips, keep the shoulders relaxed and down.

arm floats
Beginner

Objectives: To strengthen shoulder stability and to mobilize the shoulder joint.

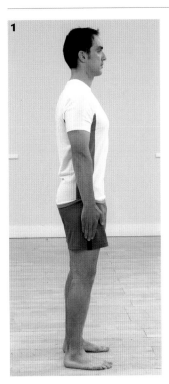
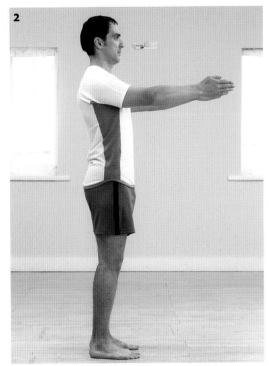

Start Position

- Start in the standing set position.

Technique

1 Breathe in to prepare
2 Breathe out and engage the Transverse Abdominus and pelvic floor muscles. Stabilize the shoulders and raise the arms, leading with the thumbs to shoulder height.
3 Breathe in to return the arms down by your side.

Repetitions

- 5–10 times

Hints & Tips

- Keep the shoulders down as your raise your arms.
- Don't lean back.
- Don't allow the ribs to flare or rise when lifting the arms.
- Keep the weight central in the feet and equally distributed.
- Imagine you have helium balloons attached to the thumbs. Let them rise effortlessly.

standing twist
Beginner

Objectives: To mobilize the thoracic spine during rotation while maintaining stability and length, strengthen trunk stability, and to develop core strength.

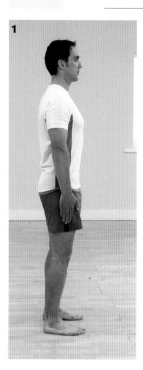

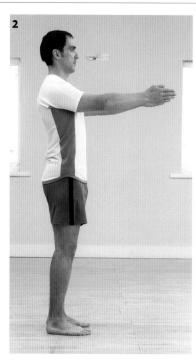

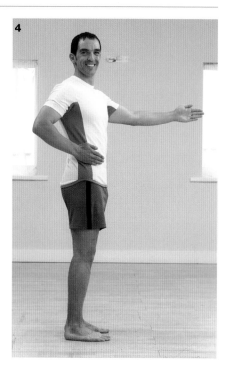

Start Position

- Start in the standing set position.

Technique

1 Breathe in to prepare.

2 Breathe out and engage the Transverse Abdominus and pelvic floor muscles, while raising the arms to shoulder level.

3 Breathe in and hold the position.

4 Breathe out and engage the Transverse Abdominus and pelvic floor muscles, drawing the right elbow in toward the waist and rotating the body to the right, looking toward the right. Keep the hip bones facing forward.

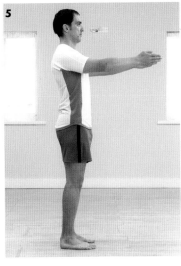

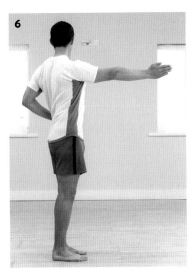

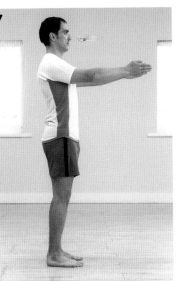

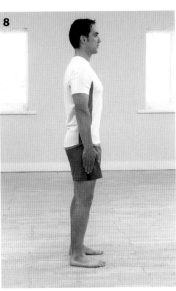

5 Breathe in to return to center.

6 Breathe out and engage the Transverse Abdominus and pelvic floor muscles, drawing the left elbow in toward the waist and rotating the body to the left, looking toward the left. Keep the hips bones facing forward.

7 Breathe out and engage the Transverse Abdominus and pelvic floor muscles and return the arms down by your side.

8 Breathe in to return to center.

Repetitions

- 5–10 times.

Hints & Tips

- Keep the hip bones facing forward during the rotation.
- Keep the shoulders down, maintaining a gap between the ear and shoulder.
- Be careful not to take the head too far around. Keep it in line with the shoulders.

63

shoulder squeeze
Beginner

Objectives: To strengthen the middle fibers of the Trapezius to encourage scapula retraction, helping to strengthen shoulder stability. To strengthen the external rotators which help to keep good upper body posture. To lengthen the chest muscles (shoulder protractors).

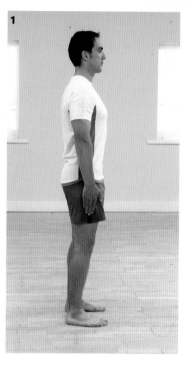 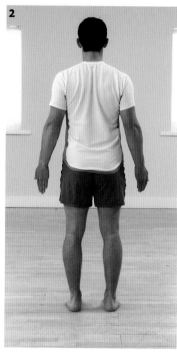 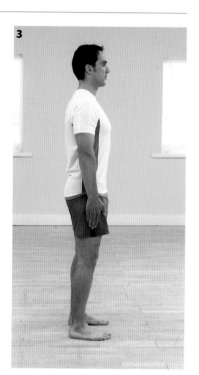

Start Position

• Start in the standing set position.

Technique

1 Breathe in to prepare.

2 Breathe out and engage the Transverse Abdominus and pelvic floor muscles. Squeeze the shoulder blades toward one another. The arms and hands will rotate as you do this.

3 Breathe in to relax the shoulder blades allowing the arms to relax and hands face the body again.

Repetitions

• 5–10 times.

Hints & Tips

• Initiate the movement from the shoulder blades, don't just move the arms.
• Keep the rib cage down during the squeeze.
• Keep a good gap between the ears and shoulders.

half roll down
Beginner

Objectives: Segmental control of the spine. To strengthen the trunk stabilizers and increase strength of the shoulder stabilizers.

1

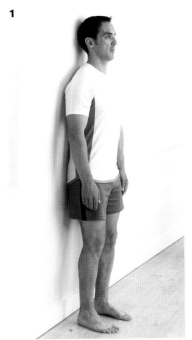

2

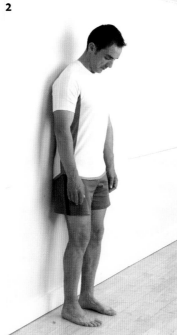

4

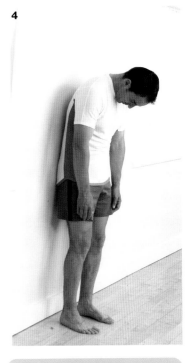

Start Position

- Start in the standing set position with your back against a wall or door.

Technique

1. Breathe in to prepare.
2. Breathe out and engage the Transverse Abdominus and pelvic floor muscles and drop your chin toward your chest, keeping your back against the wall.

3. Breathe in and hold the position.
4. Breathe out and check the Transverse Abdominus and pelvic floor muscles are engaged and peel your shoulders off the wall toward your shoulder blades.

Hints & Tips

- The roll down initially needs to be done against the wall to improve body awareness, especially if the upper body is over rounded. The idea of rolling down may seem strange as it encourages the body into a forward flexion position, which is exactly what we are trying to correct in a kyphotic posture. However, the emphasis is on the return from the roll down to the start position, which focuses our attention instead on strengthening the fibers that help us to stand up straight.

65

half roll down (continued)

5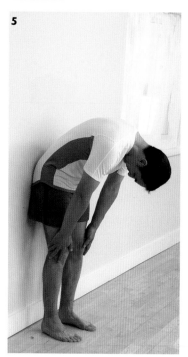

7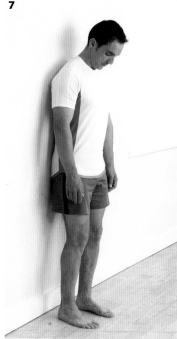

8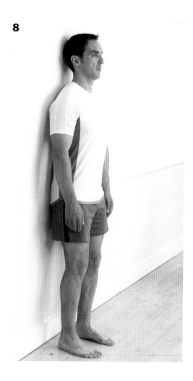

5 You can progress moving further down to your waist, if you have the flexibility.

6 Breathe in and hold the position.

7 Breathe out and re-stack your spine back up to a full standing position. Initiate the movement by drawing your shoulder blades down your back.

8 Breathe in and prepare to roll down again.

Repetitions

• 5–10 times.

Hints & Tips

• Don't allow the buttocks to come off the wall when bending forward.
• Keep your knees soft. Remember the key part of the exercise is in the re-stacking.

full roll down
Intermediate

Objectives: Segmental control of the spine. Functional movement to get from standing to the floor safely.

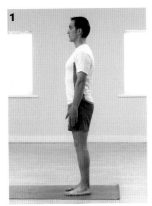
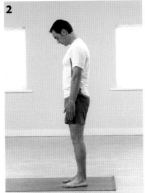
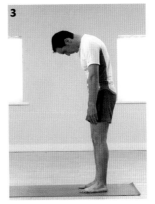

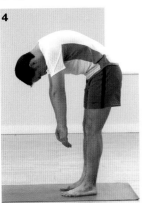
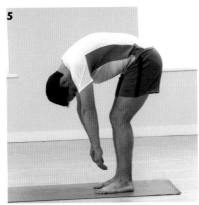

Start Position

- Start in the standing set position.

Technique

1 Breathe in to prepare.

2 Breathe out and engage the Transverse Abdominus and pelvic floor muscles. Drop the chin toward the chest.

3 Begin to slowly roll down.

4 Soften the knees, keep the Transverse Abdominus muscles engaged, and continue to breathe on the way down. Don't hold the breath.

5 Continue rolling down as far as you can comfortably go.

6 Bend the knees to get your chest to your thighs, head to knees, and your hands to the floor.

7 Bring yourself into the all fours set position.

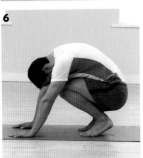
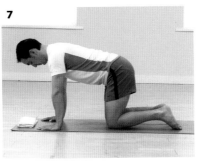

67

cat pedals
Beginner

Objectives: To strengthen all trunk stabilizers focusing mainly on shoulder stability. To develop core strength. To strengthen the spinal extensors and to encourage balance and strength.

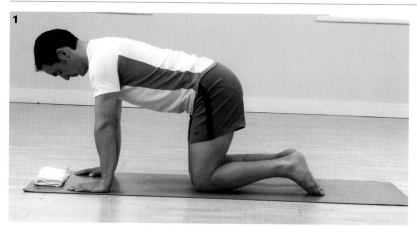

Start Position

- Start in the all fours set position, your feet apart in line with your knees.
- Your knees are in line with your hip bones, your pelvis in its neutral position.
- Engage the Transverse Abdominus muscles.
- Your rib cage is soft and down.
- Your shoulders are away from your ears and your hands in line with the shoulders.
- Keep your shoulder blades down and engaged.
- Tuck your chin in and keep your neck long.
- Breathe in and breathe out.
- Keep the pelvic floor engaged.

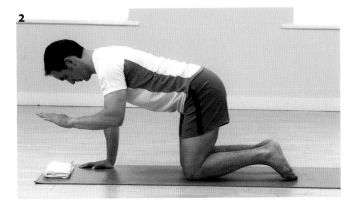

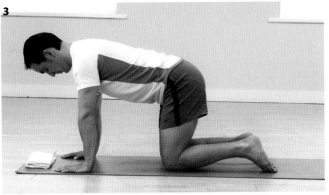

Technique

1 Breathe in to prepare.

2 Breathe out and engage the Transverse Abdominus and pelvic floor muscles. Raise one hand off the floor bending at the elbow to stop any movement occurring in the shoulders.

3 Breathe in and place the hand back on the floor.

4 Breathe out and engage the Transverse Abdominus and pelvic floor muscles and raise the other hand off the floor.

5 Breathe in to place the hand back on the floor.

Repetitions

• 2–5 times each arm then return to floor to rest the wrists.

side pocket
Beginner

Start Position

- Start in the all fours set position.

Technique

1 Breathe in to prepare.
2 Breathe out and engage the Transverse Abdominus and pelvic floor muscles. Raise the elbow past the waist, skimming the side of the body and placing the hand into an imaginary side pocket.
3 Breathe in and replace the hand on the floor.

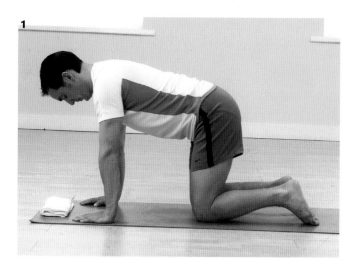

Repetitions

- 2–5 times each arm then return to floor to rest the wrists.

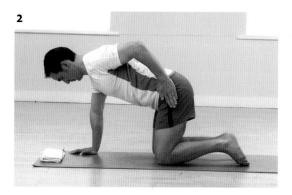

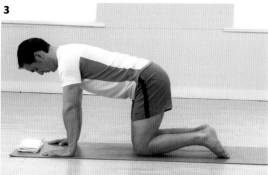

shake hands
Intermediate

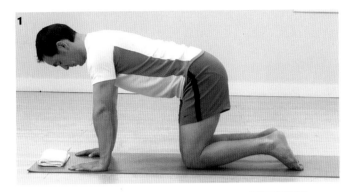

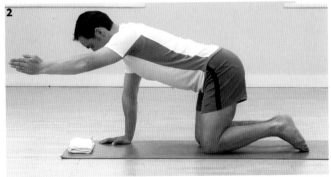

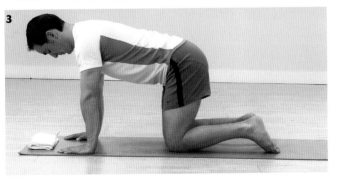

Start Position

- Start in the all fours set position.

Technique

1 Breathe in to prepare.
2 Breathe out and engage the Transverse Abdominus and pelvic floor muscles. Lengthen one arm out in front, thumbs leading the way, and keeping the shoulders away from the ears.
3 Breathe in to return the hand to the floor.

Repetitions

- 2–5 times each arm then return to floor to rest the wrists.

toe pointing
Beginner

Objectives: To strengthen all trunk stabilizers, focusing mainly on core strength and pelvic stability. To develop balance and strength.

Start Position

- The all fours set position.

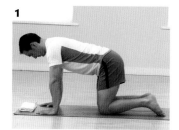
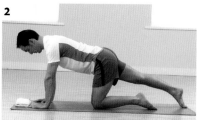
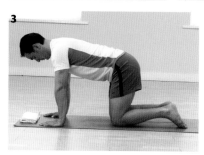

Technique

1 Breathe in to prepare.
2 Breathe out and engage the Transverse Abdominus and pelvic floor muscles. Lengthen one leg out behind, keeping the toe on the floor.
3 Breathe in to return the knee under hip.
4 Breathe out to engage Transverse Abdominus and pelvic floor. Lengthen other leg out behind, keeping toe on floor.
5 Breathe in to return knee under hip.

Repetitions

- 2–5 times on each side then rest the wrists.

Modifications
- The toe pointing exercise can be made more difficult by lifting the leg off the floor, instead of just pointing the toe. These are known as leg raises.
- Start in the all four set position.
- Breathe in to prepare.
- Breathe out and engage the Transverse Abdominus and pelvic floor muscles. Stabilize the shoulders and lengthen one leg out behind to toe point then raise the leg off the floor, maintaining a neutral pelvis.
- Breathe in to return the knee under the hip.
- Breathe out and engage the Transverse Abdominus and pelvic floor muscles. Stabilize the shoulders and lengthen the other leg out behind, pointing the toe, then raise the leg off the floor maintaining a neutral pelvis.
- Breathe in to return the knee under the hip.
- Repeat 2–5 times on each side then rest the wrists.

Hints & Tips
- Lower back does not arch when lifting leg off floor.
- Don't sink into the opposite hip.

all fours balance
Intermediate

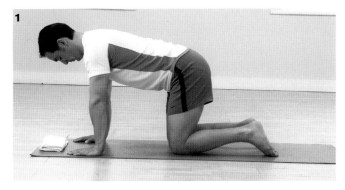

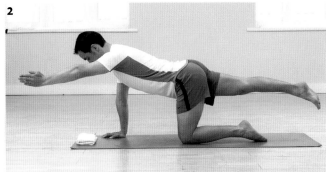

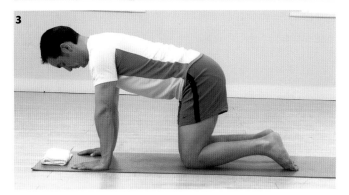

Start Position

- The all fours set position.

Technique

1 Breathe in to prepare.
2 Breathe out and engage the Transverse Abdominus and pelvic floor muscles. Stabilize the shoulders and stretch out an opposite arm to leg, maintaining a neutral pelvis.
3 Breathe in to return to the all fours position.

Repetitions

- 3–5 times alternating sides

Hints & Tips

- Keep a full spinal alignment during the movements.
- Take a rest whenever needed, as it is tiring on the wrists.
- Keep your head up in alignment with the shoulders, as it tends to drop forward in this position.

shell stretch
Beginner

Objective: To stretch and release the spinal muscles.

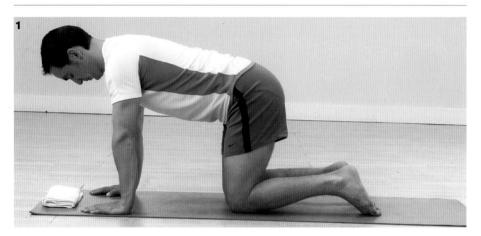

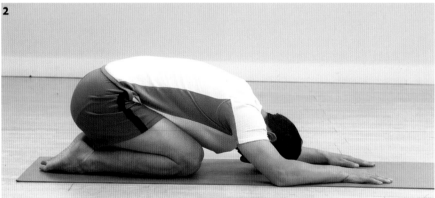

Start Position

• Start in the all fours set position.

Technique

1 Breathe in to prepare.
2 Breathe out and engage the Transverse Abdominus and pelvic floor muscles. Sit your buttocks back toward the heels and stay for 3–5 breaths.

Hints & Tips

• Use the shell stretch during the all fours exercises at any time you need to relax the wrists.
• If this causes problems in your knees, lie on your side and hug your knees in toward the chest or lie on your back and hug the knees into the chest. Either way you will release the back.

breast stroke preparation
Beginner

Objectives: To develop correct scapula stabilization by strengthening the postural muscles in the upper back. To encourage thoracic extension. To lengthen the chest muscles and strengthen the deep neck flexors.

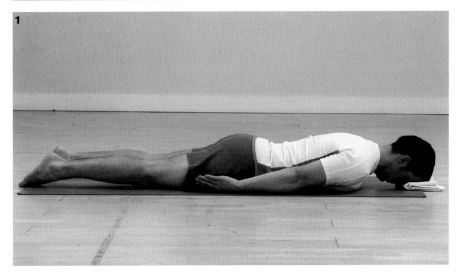

Modification

• If you find it difficult to lie on your front or get a lot of tension in your neck, shoulders, or back, then the shoulder squeeze can be done instead of breast stroke preparation. The shoulder squeeze targets the same muscles (see page 64).

Start Position

• Start in the prone set position.

• Keep your feet apart in line with your knees.

• Keep your knees in line with your hips.

• Your pelvis should be in its neutral position.

• Engage your Transverse Abdominus muscles.

• Your rib cage is soft and down.

• Your shoulders are away from the ears and your arms by your side.

• Your shoulder blades are down and engaged.

• Tuck your chin in and keep the neck long.

• Breathe in and breathe out.

• Keep your pelvic floor muscles engaged.

breast stroke preparation (continued)

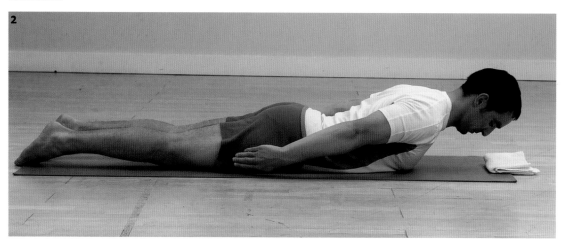

Technique

1 Breathe in to prepare.

2 Breathe out and engage the Transverse Abdominus and pelvic floor muscles. Draw the shoulder blades down the back and let the breast bone lift off the floor.

3 Breathe in.

4 Breathe out to release back to the floor.

Hints & Tips

- Omit the lift of the breast bone if it causes too much tension in the neck, shoulders, or back. Just engage the shoulder blades, raising the arms off the floor to sit at the side of the body and then release them again.
- Don't be tempted to just raise the head, initiate the movement from the shoulder blades.
- Keep the buttocks and legs relaxed throughout. If the buttocks do not relax, try doing the exercise with the feet in a pigeon toe position.

Repetitions

- 5–10 times.

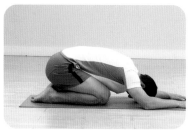

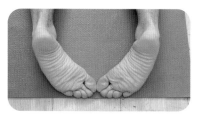

Modifications
- Pigeon toes can help to disengage activity in the gluteals and legs.
- If you experience pinching in the lower back try placing a towel under the hips.
- Add a shell stretch here if you feel a need to stretch the back out.

prone squeeze
Beginner

Objectives: To strengthen the gluteal muscles (buttocks) and hamstrings. To strengthen core stability. To develop hip mobility.

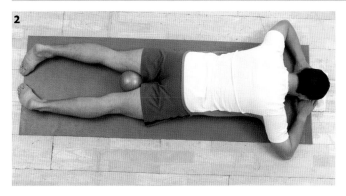

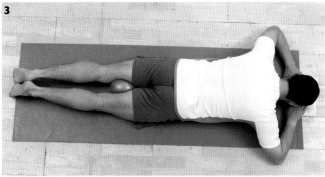

Start Position

- Start in the prone position with your feet turned in (pigeon toes), hands resting under the forehead, and shoulders stable.

Technique

1 Breathe in to prepare.
2 Place a soft ball or cushion between the top of the legs.
3 Breathe out and engage the Transverse Abdominus and pelvic floor muscles. Bring your heels together and squeeze the ball between your thighs.
4 Breathe in and allow your heels to drop apart and relax.

Repetitions

- Repeat 5–10 times.

Hints & Tips
- The hip bones and the pubic bone stay down on the floor during the movement.
- The back stays stable and in neutral.
- Keep the shoulders relaxed and down.
- Maintain the pelvic floor lift on the squeeze.

side lying open door
Beginner

Objectives: To develop thoracic rotation. To strengthen shoulder stability. To stretch the chest muscle and strengthen internal and external obliques.

Start Position

- Start in the side lying set position. (Place a block under your head for alignment and comfort.)
- Your feet are together in line with your knees.
- Knees slightly lower than hip level.
- Your pelvis is in its neutral position.
- Engage the Transverse Abdominus muscles.
- Your rib cage is soft and down.
- Keep your shoulders away from the ears and your arms out in front in line with your shoulders.
- Your shoulder blades are down and engaged.
- Tuck your chin in and keep your neck long.
- Breathe in and breathe out.
- Keep your pelvic floor muscles engaged.

Technique

1 Breathe in to prepare.
2 Breathe out and engage the Transverse Abdominus and pelvic floor muscles and raise the arm toward the ceiling, turning the head to follow the hand.
3 Breathe in.
4 Breath out and engage the Transverse Abdominus and pelvic floor muscles and close the arm following the hand with the head. Remember, the movement is just the shoulders and head, not the trunk.

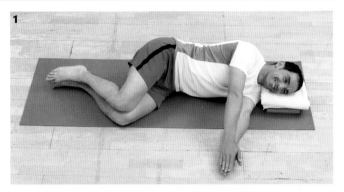

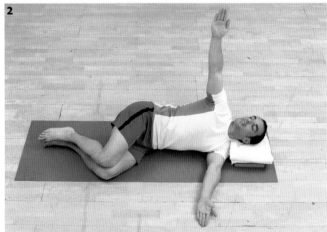

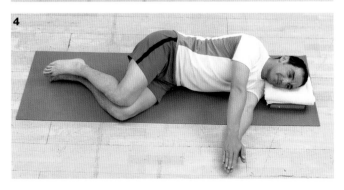

side lying open door
Intermediate

Objectives: To further develop thoracic rotation. To strengthen shoulder stability. To stretch the chest muscle and strengthen internal and external obliques.

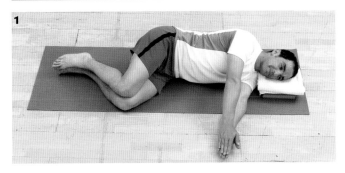

Start Position

- Start in the side lying set position. (Place a block under your head for alignment and comfort.)

Technique

1. Breathe in to prepare.
2. Breathe out and engage your Transverse Abdominus and pelvic floor muscles and raise the arm toward the ceiling, turning the head to follow the hand.
3. Breathe in and stabilize the shoulder by dropping it toward the floor.
4. Breathe out, maintaining the engagement in the Transverse Abdominus and pelvic floor muscles, and twisting from the waist to open the chest. Follow the hand with the head, keeping the knees together and the hips stacked.
5. Breathe in and hold the position.

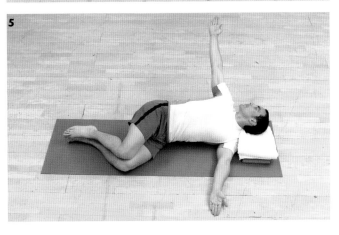

Hints & Tips

- Remember, less is more.
- Keep your hips and knees together during the movement to keep the pelvis in alignment.
- If you have stiffness in the neck, watch you only go as far as you can keeping the nose in line.
- Initiate the twist from the waist (Oblique muscle) in both directions not from the shoulders.

79

side lying open door (continued)

6 Breathe out, maintaining the engagement in the Transverse Abdominus and pelvic floor muscles, and twist from the waist to return to the side position, arm toward the ceiling.

7 Close the arm up.

Repetitions

• 5 times is all that is required if done correctly. Repeat on the other side.

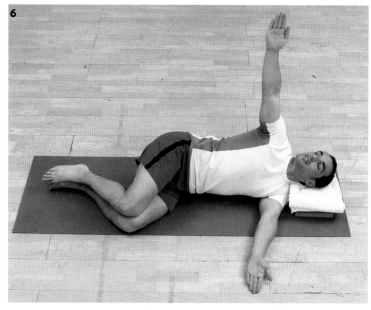

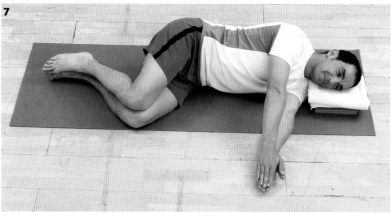

skull rock
Beginner

Objectives: To lengthen the neck extensors (nape of neck) and strengthen the neck flexors (throat). To relax the fibers in the upper Trapezius around the neck and shoulders.

Start Position

- Start in the supine set position, feet apart in line with your knees.
- Your knees are in line with your hip bones.
- Your pelvis is in its neutral position.
- Engage the Transverse Abdominus muscles.

- Your rib cage is soft and down.
- Keep your shoulders away from your ears, arms by your side.
- Keep your shoulder blades down.
- Tuck your chin in and keep your neck long.
- Breathe in and breathe out.
- Your pelvic floor is engaged.

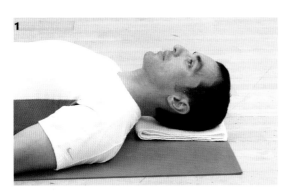 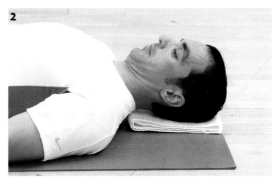

Technique

1 Breathe in to prepare.
2 Breathe out and engage the Transverse Abdominus and pelvic floor, dropping your chin toward the chest.
3 Breathe in and hold.
4 Breathe out to release your head back to its natural placement.

Repetitions

- 5–10 times.

Hints & Tips
- Don't force the chin down, keep the movement subtle.
- Keep your shoulders relaxed.

81

hamstring stretch
Beginner

Objectives: To lengthen the hamstrings. To develop core stability. To strengthen trunk stability.

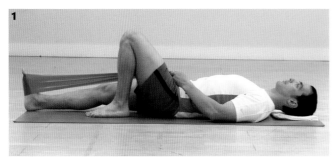

Start Position

- Start in the supine position with one leg extended. Place an exercise band or long scarf around the extended leg with your shoulders relaxed and elbows down.

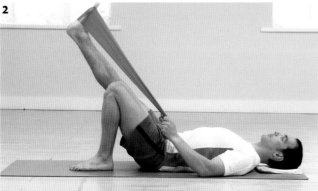

Technique

1 Breathe in to prepare.

2 Breathe out and engage the Transverse Abdominus and pelvic floor muscles, raising the leg toward the ceiling, maintaining a neutral alignment in the spine.

3 Breathe in and out and hold for 3–5 breaths.

4 Breathe in to prepare to lower the leg.

5 Breathe out and engage the Transverse Abdominus and pelvic floor muscles, lowering the leg to the floor. Relax.

Repetitions

- 3–5 on each leg.

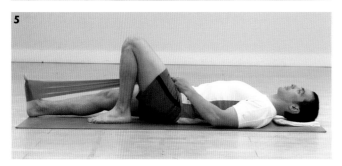

Hints & Tips

- Keep the pelvis in its neutral position.
- Keep the buttocks on the floor.
- Your shoulders are relaxed.
- Tuck your chin in slightly to keep the length in the back of the neck.

double arm circles
Beginner

Objectives: To develop good shoulder mobility and movement within the shoulder girdle. To strengthen shoulder stability.

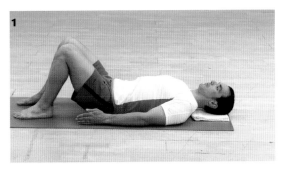

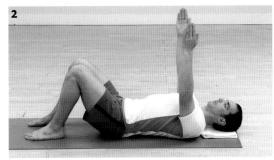

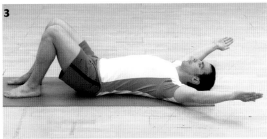

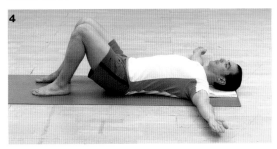

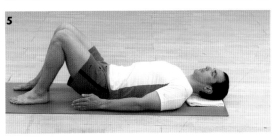

Start Position

- The supine set position.

Technique

1 Breathe in to prepare.
2 Breathe out to engage Transverse Abdominus and pelvic floor. Keep shoulders stable and head still. Start to raise the arms.
3 Breathe in and continue to raise the arms up and over the head.
4 Breathe out and engage the Transverse Abdominus and pelvic floor muscles and rotate the arms around.
5 Bring your arms back to your side.

Repetitions

- 5–10 times.

Hints & Tips
- The ribs stay down during the movement.
- The spine remains in neutral.
- Reduce the range of movement or bring the arms higher off the ground to make the movement smooth and effortless.

shoulder bridge
Intermediate

Objectives: Segmental control of the spine to increase mobility. To develop core strength, strengthen gluteals and hamstrings, strengthen trunk stability, and lengthen hip flexors.

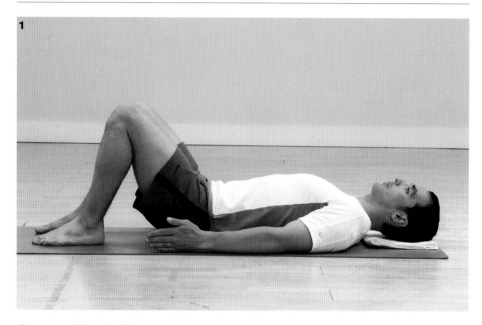

Start Position

- Start in the supine set position, with your feet a little closer to the buttocks than you would do normally.

Technique

1 Breathe in to prepare.
2 Breathe out and engage the Transverse Abdominus muscles and pelvic floor.
3 Tilt the pelvis, squeeze the buttocks, and lift off the floor, peeling one vertebrae off at a time toward the shoulder blades.

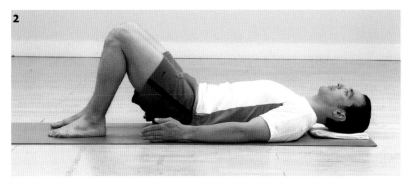

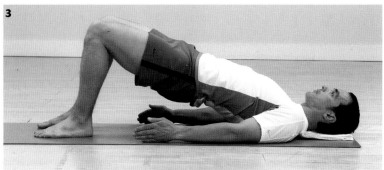

4 Breathe in and hold.

5 Breathe out and engage the Transverse Abdominus and pelvic floor muscles and return to the floor sequentially, returning the spine to neutral.

Repetitions

• Start with 5 and increase to 10

Hints & Tips

• It is a slow exercise so take as many breaths as you need to but keep checking that the abdominals are hollowed and the pelvic floor engaged. (As a rule of thumb, stop to take a breath in and continue on the out breath.)

• Check the weight distribution between your feet to see if you are favoring one side at any time.

• Only ever go up as high as is comfortable.

• Don't allow the ribs to flare as you get higher off the floor.

hip flexor stretch
Beginner

Objectives: To lengthen the hip flexor muscle, which, if tight, has a direct effect on the positioning of the pelvis.

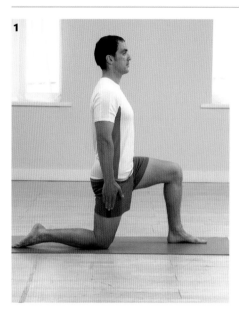

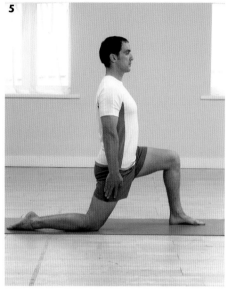

Modification
- If you find it difficult kneeling, try the alternative hip flexor stretch on page 55.

Start Position

- Kneeling with one leg out in front, knee bent at a 90-degree angle in line with ankle, back knee in line with hip.

Technique

1 Breathe in to prepare.
2 Breathe out, engage Transverse Abdominus and pelvic floor. Tuck tail bone under until you feel a mild tension in the leg you are kneeling on.

3 Hold for 3–5 breathes.
4 Relax and repeat before changing leg.
5 To progress this stretch take the knee a little further back behind the hip line.

Hints & Tips
- Don't let the back arch.
- Keep the shoulders over the hips while tucking the tail bone under.

monkey squat
Beginner

Objectives: To develop correct lifting technique and strengthen trunk stabilizers, gluteals, legs, and ankles.

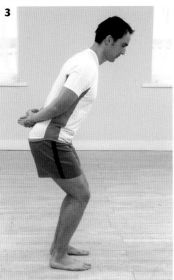

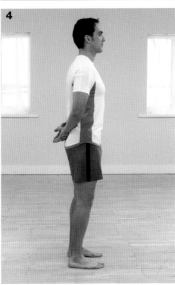

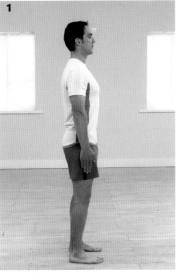

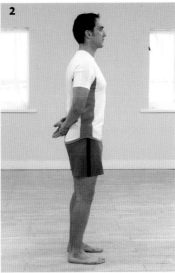

Start Position

- Standing set position, with feet apart in line with your knees.
- Knees in line with your hip bones.
- Pelvis in its neutral position.
- Transverse Abdominus slightly tensed.
- Rib cage soft and down.
- Shoulders away from the ears, arms by your side.
- Shoulder blades down and engaged.
- Chin down, neck long.
- Breathing in and out.
- Pelvic floor engaged.

Technique

1 Breathe in to prepare.
2 Place hands behind your back.
3 Breathe out to engage Transverse Abdominus and pelvic floor and hinge from the hip, bending the knees taking the bottom back. Keep the shoulders in line with the knees and the alignment in the spine.
4 Breathe in to stand.

Repetitions

- 5–10 times.

87

monkey squat
Intermediate

Objectives: To develop correct lifting technique and to strengthen trunk stabilizers, gluteals, legs, and ankles.

Start Position

• Standing set position.

Technique

1 Breathe in to prepare.
2 Breathe out and engage Transverse Abdominus and pelvic floor. Stabilize the shoulders. Hinge from the hips and bend the knees allowing the arms to fall toward the knees.
3 Breathe in to stand.

Repetitions

• 5–10 times.

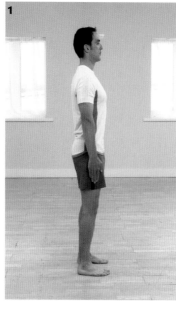

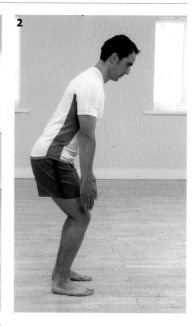

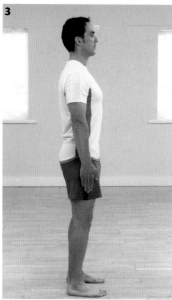

Hints & Tips

• Keep arms relaxed, they should hang from the shoulders without tension.
• The shoulder blades stay engaged to keep the chest open and lifted.
• Watch yourself in the mirror and compare your own back with the picture.

monkey squat
Advanced

Objectives: To develop correct lifting technique and strengthen the gluteals, legs, and ankles.

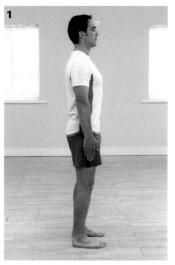

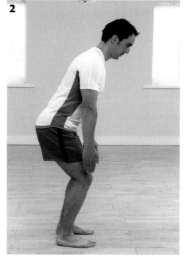

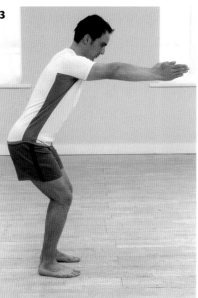

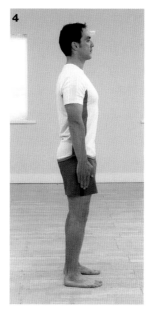

Start Position

- Standing set position.

Technique

1 Breathe in to prepare.

2 Breathe out and engage Transverse Abdominus and pelvic floor. Stabilize the shoulders. Hinge from the hips and bend at the knees, allowing the arms to fall toward the knees.

3 Raise the arms toward shoulder level, palms facing one another, fingers pointing out.

4 Breathe in to stand.

Repetitions

- 5–10 times.

Hints & Tips

- Maintain correct alignment in the spine while performing the exercise.
- Draw shoulder blades closer together whilst squatting to prevent shoulders from falling forward.

89

30-Minute Routine For Sway Back Posture Types

This routine is ideal for people who stand all day, such as shop assistants or hairdressers. It is good for those who are conscious of their height and slump and teenagers and models will also benefit from this routine.

This routine is as follows:

- Standing set position
- Standing heel raises
- Foot pedals
- Standing balance
- Arm floats
- All fours cat
- Breast stroke prep
- Prone squeeze
- Shell stretch
- Hip roll
- Hip roll intermediate
- Skull rock
- Abdominal prep
- Single leg stretch
- Single leg stretch intermediate
- Obliques
- Obliques intermediate
- Shoulder bridge
- Shoulder squeeze
- Monkey squat

standing set position
Beginner

Objectives: To develop good standing alignment and strengthen the trunk stabilizers to maintain good posture.

Start Position

- Standing set position.
- Feet apart in line with your knees.
- Knees in line with your hip bones.
- Pelvis in its neutral position.
- Transverse Abdominus slightly tensed.
- Rib cage soft and down.
- Shoulders away from the ears, arms by your side.
- Shoulder blades down and engaged.
- Chin down, neck long.
- Breathing in and out.
- Pelvic floor engaged.

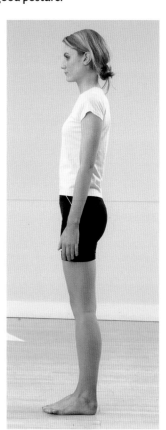

standing heel raises
Beginner

Objectives: To strengthen the Gluteal Medius muscle to help prevent the pelvis from tilting involuntarily when walking or climbing stairs. To strengthen and mobilize the ankles. To strengthen the core stabilizers. To prepare for the foot pedals and balance exercises.

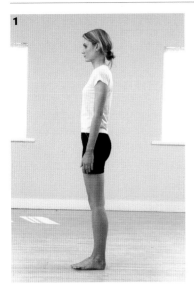

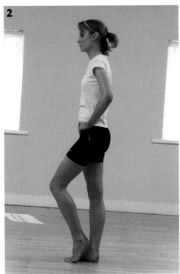

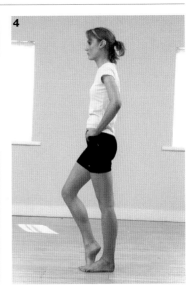

Start Position

- Standing set position.
- Feet apart in line with your knees.
- Knees in line with your hip bones.
- Pelvis in its neutral position.
- Transverse Abdominus slightly tensed.
- Rib cage soft and down.
- Shoulders away from the ears, arms by your side.
- Shoulder blades down and engaged.
- Chin down, neck long.
- Breathing in and out.
- Pelvic floor engaged.

Technique

1 Breathe in to prepare.
2 Breathe out to engage Transverse Abdominus and pelvic floor and raise the left heel away from the floor.
3 Breathe in to replace the foot down.
4 Breathe out to engage Transverse Abdominus and pelvic floor while you raise the right heel. To detect any involuntary movement in the pelvis, place the hands on the hips while you execute the moves. Your aim is to move without the pelvis rocking from side to side.
5 Breathing in to replace the foot down.

Repetitions

- 5–10 times

Hints & Tips

- Watch you don't shift your weight from one hip onto the other.
- Your weight distribution through the legs shouldn't change even as you lift the heels because the weight should just transfer into the ball of the foot.
- If you watch yourself in the mirror, you are aiming to see no movement within the body, just the legs.

foot pedals
Intermediate

Objectives: To strengthen the ankles and develop mobility. To strengthen the stability of the hips. To increase strength of the Gluteal Medius muscle, which helps to stabilize the pelvis.

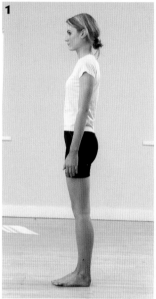

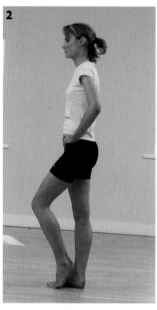

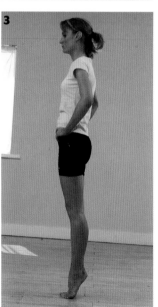

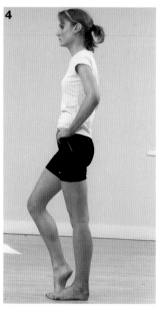

Start Position

- Standing set position with arms either by your side or resting on the hips.

Technique

1 Breathe in to prepare.
2 Breathe out to engage the Transverse Abdominus and pelvic floor and raise the left heel.
3 Breathe in to engage the Transverse Abdominus and pelvic floor and raise the right heel to balance.
4 Breathe out to lower the left heel and bend the right knee, keeping the right heel up.
5 Breathe in to raise both heels to balance.
6 Breathe out to lower, keeping the left heel up.

Repetitions

- 5–10 times depending on the strength of the ankles.

Hints & Tips

- Aim to go straight up and down rather than shifting from side to side.
- When the hands are resting on the hips, keep the shoulders relaxed and down.

standing balance
Intermediate

Objective: To strengthen the ankles and develop mobility. To strengthen the stability of the hips. To increase strength of the Gluteal Medius muscle which helps to stabilize the pelvis.

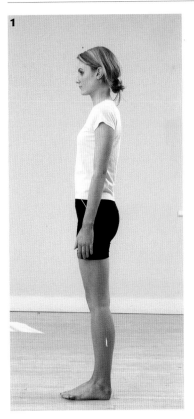

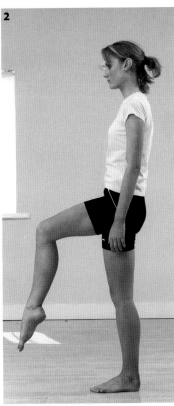

Start Position

- Standing set position.

Technique

1 Breathe in to prepare.
2 Breathe out, engage Transverse Abdominus and pelvic floor and bring one foot off the floor, raising the knee toward 90 degrees.
3 Breathe in to replace the foot down.
4 Breathe out to engage Transverse Abdominus and pelvic floor and bring the other foot off the floor, raising knee toward 90 degrees.

Repetitions

- 5–10 times.

Hints & Tips

- Keep lifted out of the hip so as not to sink or slump into opposite side.
- Keep abdominals tight to prevent leaning back.
- Place hands on hips to check stability.

93

arm floats
Beginner

Objectives: To strengthen shoulder stability. To mobilize the shoulder joint.

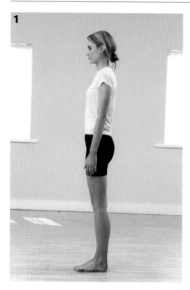

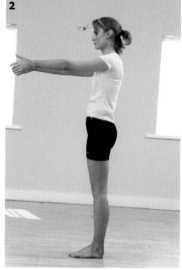

Start Position

- Standing set position.

Repetitions

- 5–10 times.

Technique

1 Breathe in to prepare.

2 Breathe out to engage Transverse Abdominus and pelvic floor. Stabilize the shoulders and raise the arms, leading with the thumbs to shoulder level. Imagine you have helium balloons attached to the thumbs, so the arms float up and float down effortlessly.

3 Breathe in to return the arms down by your side.

Hints & Tips

- Keep the shoulders down as the arms raise.
- Don't allow the ribs to flare or rise when lifting the arms.
- Keep the weight central in the feet and equally distributed.

all fours cat
Beginner

Objectives: To strengthen all trunk stabilizers focusing mainly on shoulder stability. To develop core strength and to bone load the upper body, strengthen the spinal extensors, and encourage balance and strength.

1
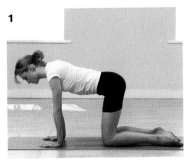
2
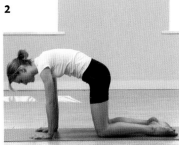
3
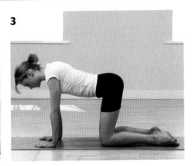

Start Position

- All fours set position.
- Feet apart in line with your knees.
- Knees in line with your hip bones.
- Pelvis in its neutral position.
- Transverse Abdominus slightly tensed.
- Rib cage soft and down.
- Shoulders away from the ears, hands directly under the shoulders.
- Shoulder blades down and engaged.
- Chin down, neck long.
- Breathing in and out.
- Pelvic floor engaged.

Technique

1 Breathe in to prepare.
2 Breathe out to engage Transverse Abdominus and pelvic floor, tuck the tail bone down and drop the head to lift up from your center, tightening the abdominals.
3 Breathe in to send tail bone toward the ceiling, allowing the back to arch gently, keeping the shoulders blades down.
4 Breathe out to engage Transverse Abdominus and pelvic floor. Stabilize shoulders and return to the all fours set position.

Repetitions

- 5–10 times.

shell stretch

1 This helps to stretch out after the all fours cat. Breathe in to sit back toward the heels.
2 Breathe out to relax and release. Give the hands a shake out.

1
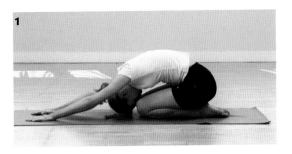

breast stroke preparation
Beginner

Objective: To develop correct scapula stabilization by strengthening the postural muscles in the upper back. To strengthen postural fibers and develop thoracic extension. To lengthen the chest muscles and to strengthen the deep neck flexors.

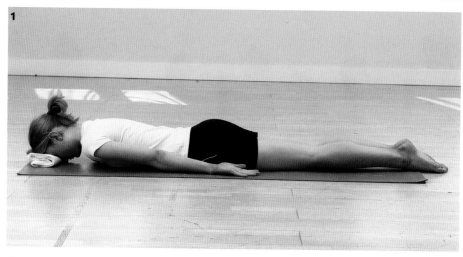

Start Position

- Prone set position.
- Feet apart in line with your knees.
- Knees in line with your hip bones.
- Pelvis in its neutral position.
- Transverse Abdominus slightly tensed.
- Rib cage soft and down.
- Shoulders away from the ears, arms by your side.
- Shoulder blades down and engaged.
- Chin down, neck long.
- Breathing in and out.
- Pelvic floor engaged.

Technique

1   Breathe in to prepare. Watch that head alignment is correct when prone.

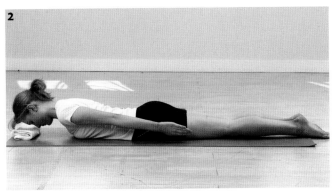

2

2 Breathe out, engage Transverse Abdominus and pelvic floor and draw the shoulder blades down into the back pockets. Lift the breast bone off the floor.

3 Breathe in.

4 Breathe out to release back to the floor.

Repetitions

• 5–10 times.

Note:

Pigeon toes (see right) can help to relax the gluteals (buttocks) and it can also help to eliminate the feeling of pinching in the lower back.

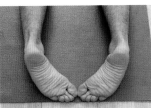

Add a shell stretch here if you feel the need to stretch out (see image on the right).

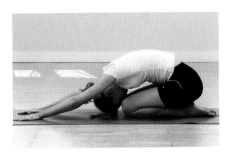

Hints & Tips

• Keep the buttocks and legs relaxed throughout.
• Don't be tempted to just raise the head, initiate the movement from the shoulder blades.

prone squeeze
Beginner

Objectives: To strengthen the gluteal muscles (buttocks) and hamstrings. To strengthen core stability and develop hip mobility.

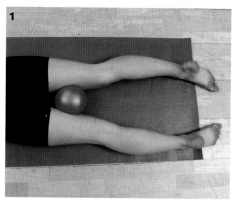

Start Position

- Prone with feet turned in (pigeon toes) and hands resting under forehead, shoulders stable.

- Place a soft ball or cushion between the top of the legs.

Technique

1 Breathe in to prepare.
2 Breathe out to engage Transverse Abdominus and pelvic floor. Bring heels together and squeeze ball between thighs.
3 Breathe in and allow heels to drop apart.

Repetitions

- 5–10 times.

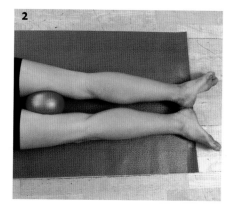

Hints & Tips

- The hip bones and the pubic bone stay down on the floor during the movement.
- The back stays stable and in neutral.
- Keep the shoulders relaxed and down.
- Maintain the pelvic floor lift on the squeeze.

shell stretch
Beginner

Objectives: To stretch and release back extensors.

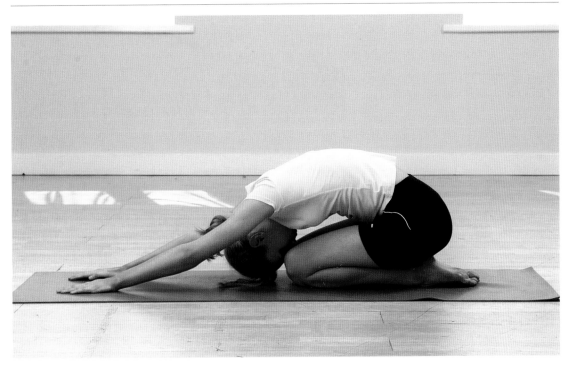

Technique

1 Breathe in and out while in this position, keeping the body relaxed.

Hints & Tips

- Knees can be quite far apart in order to get chest close to thighs.
- If you have any knee problems, roll onto back or side and hug knees into chest.

hip roll
Beginner

Objectives: To mobilize the lumbar rotators of the spine. To strengthen the trunk stabilizers and the internal and external obliques. To develop core strength.

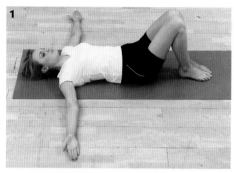

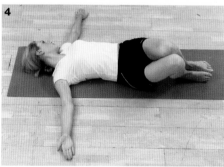

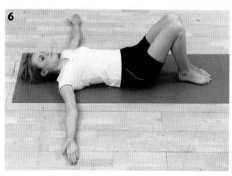

Start Position

• Supine set position with knees and feet together.

Technique

1 Breathe in to prepare.

2 Breathe out to engage Transverse Abdominus and pelvic floor.

3 Take the knees toward the right, turning the head toward the left.

4 Turn the left palm toward the floor to create stability in the shoulder leaving the right hand facing the ceiling.

5 Breathe in.

6 Breathe out to engage Transverse Abdominus and pelvic floor and bring the knees and head back to center. Focus on using the obliques in the waist when returning to center.

7 Repeat to the other side.

Repetitions

• 5–10 times.

Hints & Tips

• Keep shoulders down on the floor throughout.
• Don't take the legs too far to the side or the back will overextend causing the ribs to rise.

hip roll
Intermediate

Objectives: To lengthen and strengthen the obliques. To develop good rotation of the spine with segmental control. To promote awareness of the shoulder blades and to strengthen the shoulder stabilizers.

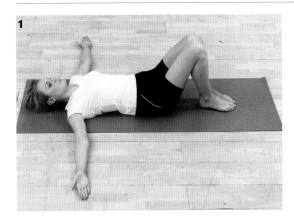

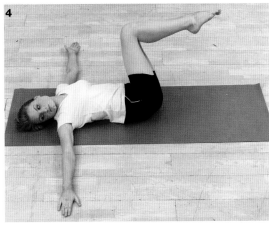

Start Position

- Supine set position.

Technique

1 Breathe in to prepare.

2 Breathe out to engage Transverse Abdominus and pelvic floor and raise one leg off the floor.

3 Breathe in to imprint the spine by pressing the low back gently toward the floor.

4 Breathe out to engage Transverse Abdominus and pelvic floor and raise the second leg without moving the spine.

5 Breathe in.

6 Breathe out, engage Transverse Abdominus and pelvic floor, and take knees to left and turn head to right.

7 Breathe in.

8 Breathe out to engage Transverse Abdominus and pelvic floor and return legs and head to center, focusing on using the obliques.

Repetitions

- 5 times on each side.

Hints & Tips

- You have to be careful that your alignment is kept in the spine and in the neck. This picture shows correct head alignment.
- Keep the awareness in the waist muscles which are initiating the movement on the return.

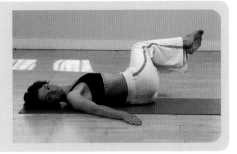

skull rock
Beginner

Objectives: To lengthen the neck extensors (nape of neck) and strengthen the neck flexors (throat). Also relaxes fibers in Upper Trapezius around the neck and shoulders.

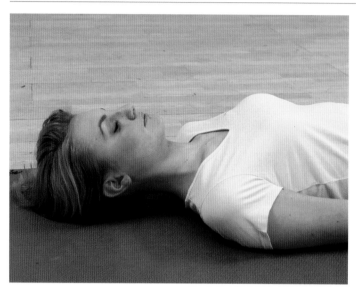

Start Position

- Supine set position.

Repetitions

- 5–10 times.

Technique

1 Breathe in to prepare.
2 Breathe out to engage Transverse Abdominus and pelvic floor. Drop chin toward the chest.
3 Breathe in.
4 Breathe out to release head back to its natural placement.

Hints & Tips
- Don't force the chin down—this is a small movement.
- Keep shoulders relaxed.

abdominal preparation
Beginner

Objectives: To strengthen the Transverse Abdominus by maintaining abdominal hollowing while lifting the head. This exercise also strengthens the core, the shoulder stabilizers, and the deep neck flexors.

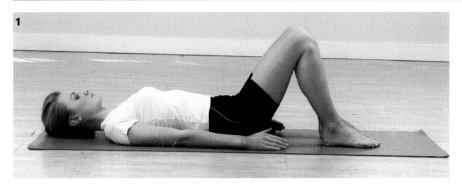

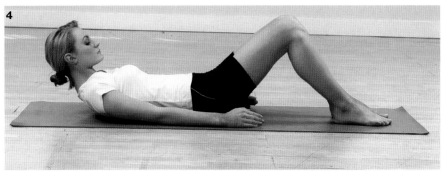

Modification
- If you suffer with neck or shoulder problems, do not lift head off the floor. Continue with everything else just omit the lifting of the head and shoulders.

Start Position

- Supine set position.

Repetitions

- Start with 5 and build up to 10 as it can be very tiring on the neck muscles.

Technique

1 Breathe in to prepare.
2 Breathe out to engage Transverse Abdominus and pelvic floor.
3 Breathe in for skull rock.
4 Breathe out to slide the ribs toward the hips, hands toward the ankles. Raise the head and the shoulders and look toward the knees.
5 Breathe in to return.
6 Breathe out to release and relax.

Hints & Tips

- Use the modification if you have any neck or shoulder problems.
- Don't raise the head and shoulders if the abdominals are doming.
- Buttocks stay relaxed.
- Pelvis stays in neutral.
- Don't forget to do the skull rock before lifting the head.

103

single leg stretch
Beginner

Objective: To develop core strength. To strengthen trunk stabilizers and increase coordination skills.

Start Position

- Supine set position.

Techniques

1 Breathe in to prepare. Do skull rock.

2 Breathe out to engage Transverse Abdominus and pelvic floor. Raise one leg off the floor.

3 Breathe in.

4 Breathe out to engage Transverse Abdominus and pelvic floor. Raise the other leg.

5 Breathe in and take hold of the left leg gently.

6 Breathe out to engage Transverse Abdominus and pelvic floor as you extend the right leg away.

7 Breathe in as the leg returns toward the chest and you swap the hands over.

8 Breathe out to engage Transverse Abdominus and pelvic floor as you extend the left leg away.

Repetitions

- 5–10 times on each leg.

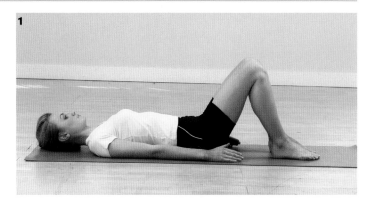

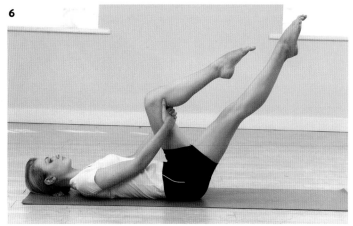

Hints & Tips

- The spine remains still and stable throughout the movement.
- Neck remains long and relaxed on the mat or your head support if using one.
- The abdominals are not to dome when the leg extends.
- The back stays down on the floor.

single leg stretch
Intermediate

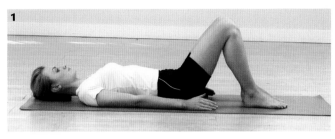

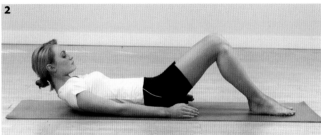

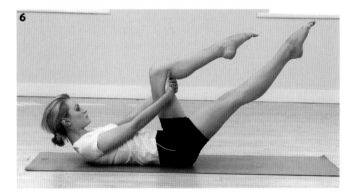

Start Position

- Supine set position.

Technique

1 Breathe in to prepare.
2 Breathe out to engage Transverse Abdominus and pelvic floor. Slide ribs to hips and raise head and shoulders to look toward the knees.
3 Breathe in to raise one leg off the floor.
4 Breathe out, engage Transverse Abdominus and pelvic floor and raise the other leg.
5 Breathe in to hold the left leg gently.
6 Breathe out to engage the Transverse Abdominus and pelvic floor as you extend the right leg away.
7 Breathe in as the leg returns toward the chest and swap the hands over.
8 Breathe out, engage Transverse Abdominus and pelvic floor as the right leg extends.

Repetitions

- 5–10 on each leg.

Hints & Tips

- Maintain neutral pelvis so the back does not arch or press down.
- If the neck begins to ache during the repetitions put it down but continue with the legs.

obliques
Beginner

Objectives: To strengthen the abdominals, focusing on the obliques (waist muscles). To develop core strength and strengthen trunk stabilizers.

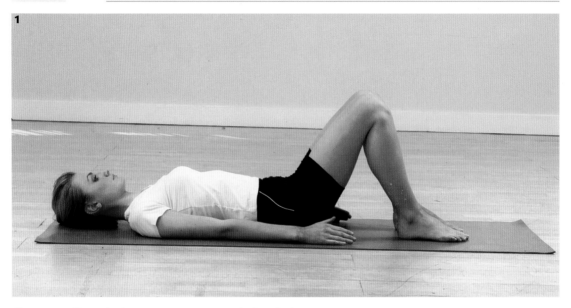

Start Position

• Supine set position.

Technique

1 Breathe in to prepare.

2 Breathe in, taking the hands behind the head.

3 Breath out to engage Transverse Abdominus and pelvic floor. Rotate the body taking the left elbow toward the ceiling, with the right elbow toward the floor. The left shoulder comes toward the right hip, raising the shoulder blade away from the floor.

4 Breathe in to return to center.

5 Breathe out to engage Transverse Abdominus and pelvic floor. Rotate the body taking the right elbow toward the ceiling, with the left elbow toward the floor. The right shoulder comes toward the left hip, raising the right shoulder blade away from the floor.

6 Breathe in to return to center.

Repetitions

• 5–10 on each side.

2

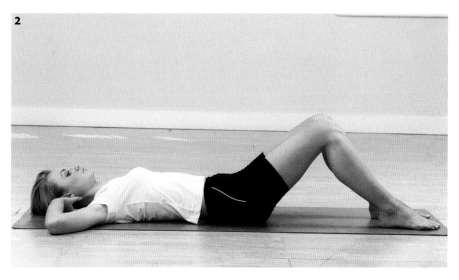

3

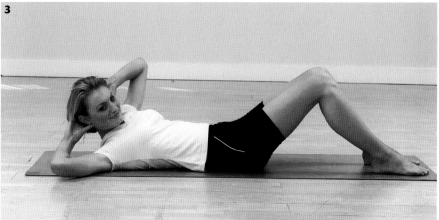

Hints & Tips

- The elbows stay wide, chest open.
- The movement is initiated in the obliques.
- Keep it small so the internal obliques are targeted rather than the external ones.

obliques with single leg stretch
Intermediate

Objectives: To increase coordination and strength in the abdominals while maintaining pelvic stability.

Start Position

- Supine set position

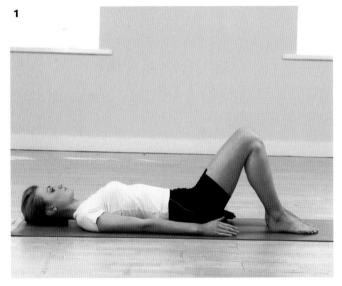

Technique

1 Breathe in to prepare for skull rock.

2 Breathe out to engage Transverse Abdominus and pelvic floor. Slide ribs to hips and raise head off the floor to look toward the knees.

3 Breathe in to raise one leg off the floor.

4 Breathe out to maintain tension in Transverse Abdominus and pelvic floor and raise other leg off the floor.

5 Breathe in and take both hands behind the head.

6 Breathe out maintain Transverse Abdominus and pelvic floor as you extend the left leg away and rotate the left shoulder toward the right knee, maintaining neutral pelvis.

7 Breathe in to return to center, both knees in.

8 Breathe out to maintain Transverse Abdominus and pelvic floor. Extend the right leg away and rotate the right shoulder toward the left knee.

9 Breathe in to center.

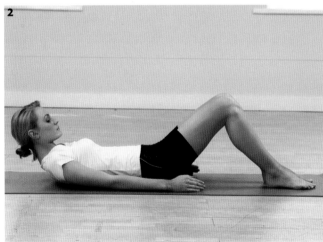

Repetitions

- 5–10 times on each leg.

Note:

This exercise requires strong abdominals in order for it to be executed correctly.

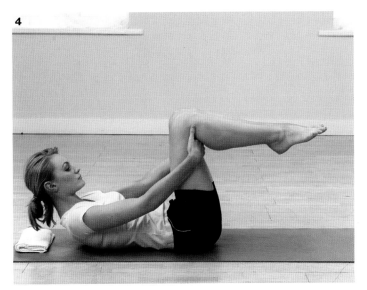

4

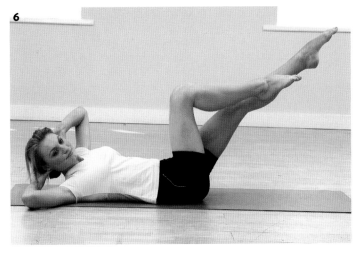

6

Hints & Tips

- Don't rock in the pelvis while rotating from one side to the other.
- Abdominals stay hollowed—no doming.
- Elbows stay wide, chest open.
- Don't pull on head or neck.

109

shoulder bridge
Intermediate

Objectives: To improve segmental control of the spine to increase mobility. To develop core, strengthen gluteals and hamstrings, improve trunk stability, and lengthen hip flexors.

Start Position

• Supine set position. Feet a little closer to the buttocks than you would have them normally. If you have been using a block under your head in this position, take it away for this exercise only.

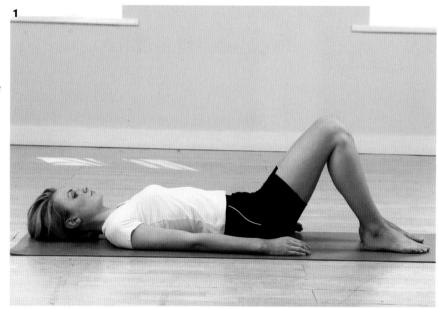

Technique

1 Breathe in to prepare.

2 Breathe out to engage Transverse Abdominus and pelvic floor. Tilt the pelvis.

3 Breathe in.

4 Breathe out to maintain Transverse Abdominus and pelvic floor. Squeeze the buttocks and lift off the floor, peeling one vertebrae off at a time, lifting toward the shoulder blades.

5 Breathe in.

6 Breathe out to engage Transverse Abdominus and pelvic floor. Go down to the floor sequentially, returning the spine to neutral.

Repetitions

• Start with 5 and increase to 10.

2

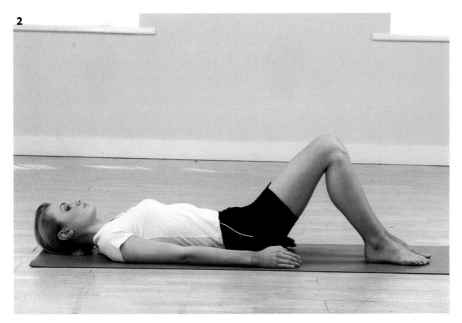

4

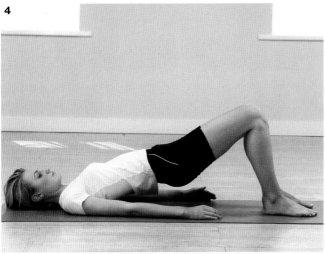

Hints & Tips

- It is a slow exercise so take as many breaths as you need.
- Keep checking that the abdominals are hollowed and the pelvic floor engaged.
- Check the weight distribution between your feet to see if you are favoring one side at any time.
- Only ever go up as high as comfortable.
- Don't allow the ribs to flare as you get higher off the floor.

shoulder squeeze
Beginner

Objectives: This exercise strengthens the middle fibers of the Trapezius to encourage scapula retraction. This helps to strengthen shoulder stability and the external rotators which help to keep good upper body posture and lengthen the chest muscles.

Start Position

- Standing set position.
- Feet apart in line with your knees.
- Knees in line with your hip bones.
- Pelvis in its neutral position.
- Transverse Abdominus slightly tensed.
- Rib cage soft and down.
- Shoulders away from the ears, arms by your side.
- Shoulder blades down and engaged.
- Chin down, neck long.
- Breathe in and out.
- Pelvic floor engaged.

Technique

1 Breathe in to prepare.
2 Breathe out to engage Transverse Abdominus and pelvic floor. Squeeze the shoulder blades toward one another and the arms and hands will rotate out.
3 Breathe in to relax the shoulder blades, allowing the arms to relax and hands face the body again.

Repetitions

- 5–10 times.

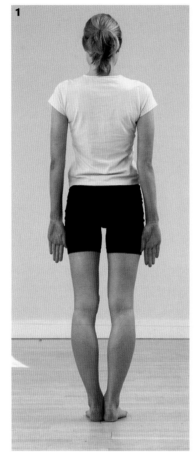
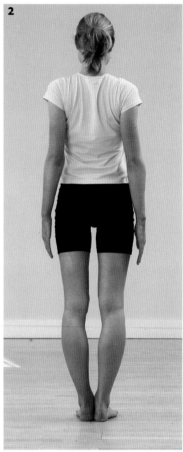

Hints & Tips

- Initiate the movement from the shoulder blades, don't just move the arms.
- Keep the rib cage down during the squeeze.
- Keep a good gap between ear and shoulder.

monkey squat
Beginner

Objectives: To develop correct lifting skills by strengthening trunk stabilizers whilst bending. To strengthen the gluteal, legs, and ankles.

Start Position

• Standing set position.

Technique

1 Breathe in to prepare.

2 Breathe out to engage Transverse Abdominus and pelvic floor. Stabilize the shoulders. Hinge from the hips and bend the knees, taking the bottom back and hands toward the knees.

3 Raise the arms toward shoulder level.

4 Breathe in to return to standing.

Repetitions

• Start with 5 and progress to 10.

Hints & Tips
• Spine stays neutral.
• Bend at the knees not the waist.
• Keep shoulders in line with the hip.
• Keep arches lifted in feet.

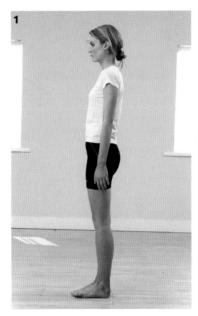

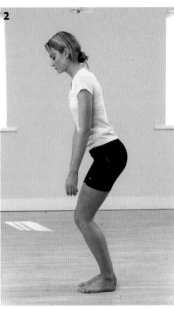

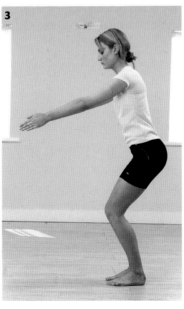

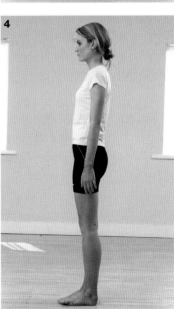

113

30-Minute Routine For Flat Backs

The exercises in this routine are designed for a flat back but can be grouped together with the kyphotic routine if you sit for prolonged periods during the day or know that you tend to slouch when sitting. Stiffness in the low back is a problem with flat back postures and therefore extra care needs to be taken when trying to mobilize areas that are fixed.

This routine is as follows:

- Arm floats
- Standing heel raises
- Foot pedals
- Roll down
- Roll down intermediate
- Seated "c" curve
- Roll down advanced
- Hamstring stretch
- Shoulder bridge
- Hip roll
- Hip roll intermediate
- Abdominal preparation
- Side lying open door
- Side lying open door intermediate
- Swimming legs
- Swimming arms
- Breast stroke
- Swan dive
- Cat's tail
- Monkey squat

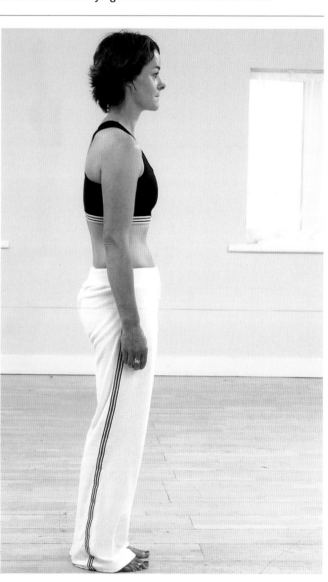

arm floats
Beginner

Objectives: To strengthen shoulder stability and to mobilize the shoulder joint.

Start Position

- Standing set position.
- Feet apart in line with your knees.
- Knees in line with your hip bones.
- Pelvis in its neutral position.
- Transverse Abdominus slightly tensed.
- Rib cage soft and down.
- Shoulders away from the ears, arms by your side.
- Shoulder blades down and engaged.
- Chin down, neck long.
- Breathing in and out.
- Pelvic floor engaged.

Technique

1 Breathe in to prepare.
2 Breathe out to engage Transverse Abdominus and pelvic floor. Stablize the shoulders and raise arms toward shoulder height.
3 Breathe in to lower the arms back down by your sides.

Repetitions

- 5–10 times.

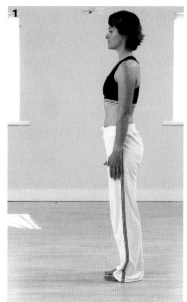

Hints & Tips

- Shoulders stay down while lifting the arms.
- Weight stays equally distributed between both feet.
- Rib cage stays down.
- Thumbs lead the way—imagine helium balloons lifting the arms so they float up.

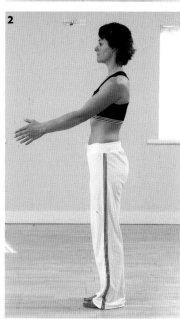

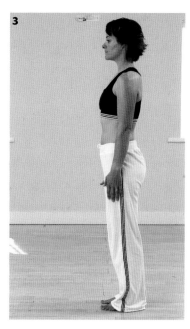

115

standing heel raises
Beginner

Objectives: To strengthen the Gluteal Medius muscle to help prevent the pelvis from tilting involuntarily when walking or climbing stairs. To strengthen and mobilize the ankles. To strengthen the core stabilizers.

Note:

This can get tiring on the ankles, especially if you have not worked them recently. The feet are always supported in shoes or trainers and we very rarely walk around in bare feet so the muscles rely on that support. When we come to work without support they fatigue quickly.

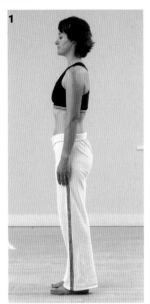
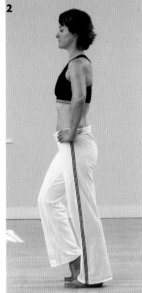
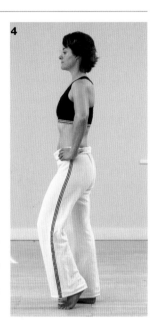

Start Position

• Standing set position.

Repetitions

• 5–10 times.

Technique

1 Breathe in to prepare.

2 Breathe out to engage Transverse Abdominus and pelvic floor and raise one heel away from the floor.

3 Breathe in to replace the foot down.

4 Breathe out to engage Transverse Abdominus and pelvic floor while you raise the other heel. Place the hands on the hip bones to feel the movement that is happening in the pelvis while changing from leg to the other. Your aim is to feel no movement in the pelvis at all.

Hints & Tips

• Watch you don't shift your weight from one hip onto the other.
• Your weight distribution through the legs shouldn't change even as you lift the heels because the weight should just transfer into the ball of the foot.
• If you watch yourself in the mirror, you are aiming to see no movement in the body.

foot pedals
Intermediate

Objectives: To strengthen the ankles and develop mobility. To strengthen the stability of the hips. To increase strength of the Gluteal Medius muscle which helps to stabilize the pelvis.

Start Position

- Standing set position, hands down by your side or resting on the hips.

Technique

1 Breathe in to prepare.
2 Breathe out to engage the Transverse Abdominus and pelvic floor and raise the right heel.
3 Breathe in to maintain the Transverse Abdominus and pelvic floor and raise the other heel to balance.
4 Breathe out to lower the right heel and bend the left knee, keeping the left heel up. Breathe in to raise both heels to balance, breathe out to lower left heel.

Repetitions

- 5–10 times depending on the strength of the ankles.

Hints & Tips

- Look to go straight up and straight down, rather than shifting from side to side.
- Imagine you are between two planks of wood and you can only go up and down.
- When the hands are resting on the hips, keep the shoulders relaxed and down.

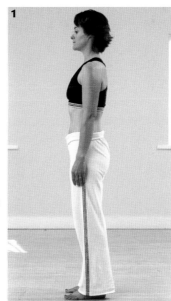
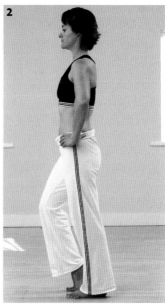
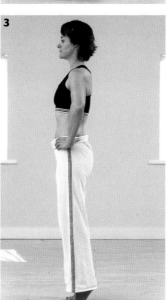
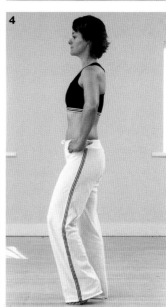

117

roll down
Beginner

Objectives: The emphasis in this exercise is to increase the mobility of the spine in areas where it is fixed. It also strengthens the trunk stabilizers.

Start Position

- Standing set position.

Technique

1 Breathe in to prepare.

2 Breathe out to engage the Transverse Abdominus and pelvic floor. Drop the chin toward the chest.

3 Take the head and shoulders a little further down toward the shoulder blades.

4 Breathe in.

5 Breathe out to engage Transverse Abdominus and pelvic floor and start to restack the spine back to standing.

Repetitions

- 5–10 times.

Hints & Tips

- At this level watch you don't hinge from the hips when taking the head and shoulders forward.
- Don't take it any further if you feel tension in the back.

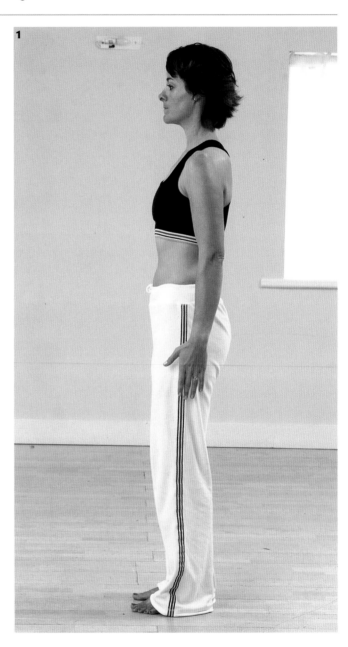

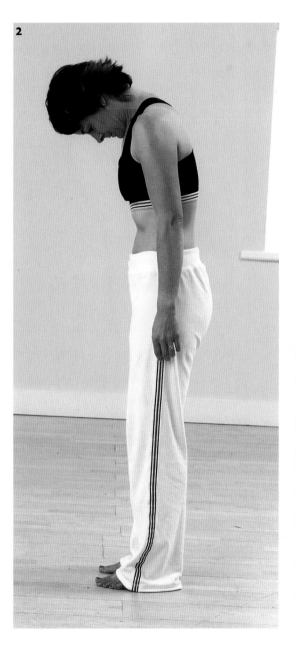

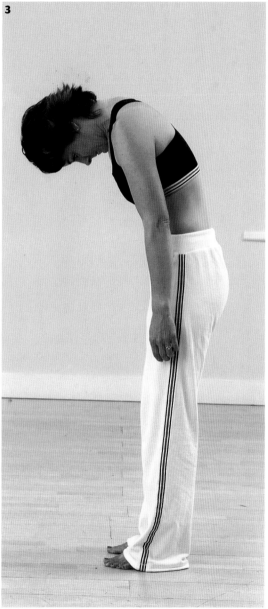

roll down
Intermediate

Objectives: To increase the mobility of the spine in areas where it is fixed.

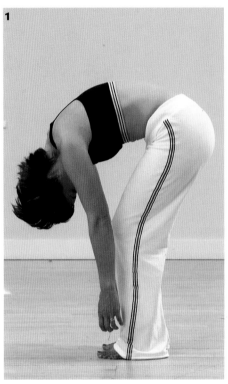

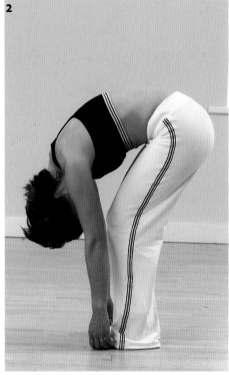

Start Position

• Standing set position.

Technique

1 Taking the roll down a little further, bending at the knees as you get further toward the floor, maintaining abdominal hollowing to support the lower back.

2 Position yourself chest to thigh, head to knee, and hands to the floor.

3 Breathe in.

4 Breathe out to start restacking the spine.

5 Move from the tail bone, sending it toward the floor as you stand.

6 Come back up to a full standing position.

7 Breathe in.

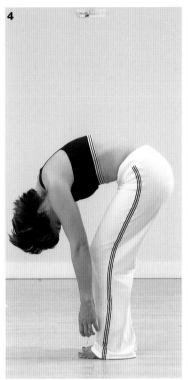

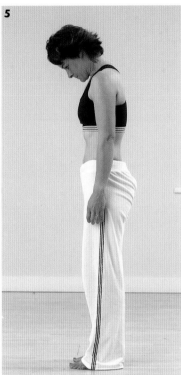

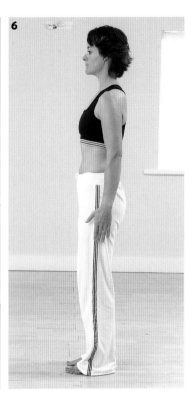

Repetitions

- 5–10 times.

Hints & Tips

- Don't hinge at the hips on roll down, bend the knees.
- Keep knees soft not locked out at any time.

seated "c" curve
Beginner

Objectives: To strengthen the abdominals and develop core strength. To mobilize and strengthen the spinal muscles. To strengthen the shoulder stabilizers while sitting.

Start Position

- Seated set position.
- If slumping use a block.
- Legs crossed or knees bent and apart.
- Knees in line with your hip bones unless crossed.
- Pelvis in its neutral position.
- Transverse Abdominus slightly tensed.
- Rib cage soft and down.
- Shoulders away from the ears, hands resting on the knees.
- Shoulder blades down and engaged.
- Chin down, neck long.
- Breathing in and out.
- Pelvic floor engaged.

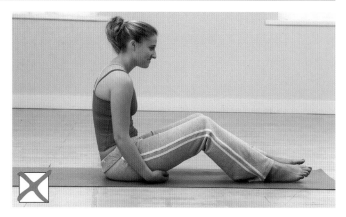

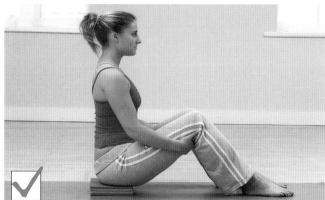

Hints & Tips
- Initiate the movement from the pelvis not the shoulders.
- The shoulders stay over the hips during the movement (ask someone to check or watch yourself side on in the mirror). There should be an imaginary line from the shoulder to side of hip when sitting upright and when in "c" curve.

Technique

1 Breathe in to prepare.

2 Breathe out to engage the Transverse Abdominus and pelvic floor, tilting the pelvis to create a "c" curve in the spine.

3 Breathe in to lift and return to neutral spine.

Repetitions

• Start with 5 and build up to 10 as this can be tiring on the hip flexors and spinal muscles.

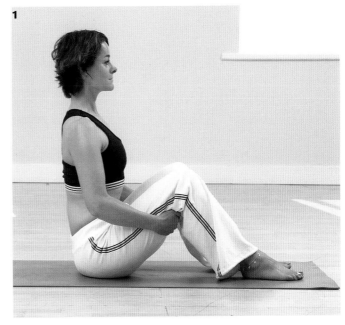

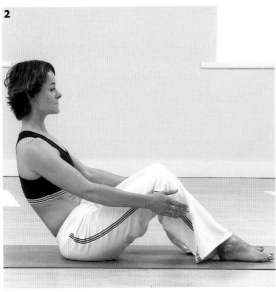

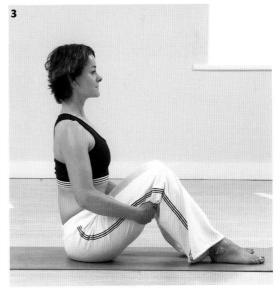

roll down
Advanced

Objectives: To strengthen abdominals while also lengthening them. To strengthen the spinal muscles during flexion. To mobilize the spine segmentally. To strengthen all torso stabilizers. To develop core strength.

Start Position

• Seated set position with knees in front.

Technique

1 Breathe in to prepare.

2 Breathe out to engage Transverse Abdominus and pelvic floor. Tilt the pelvis to create a "c" curve.

3 Continue to roll down segmentally toward the floor, keeping your feet down.

4 Breathe in to lengthen the legs away, taking the arms up and over the head.

5 Breathe in for skull rock and to raise the arms to the ceiling.

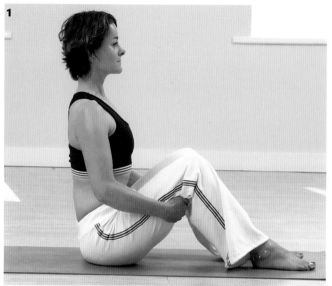

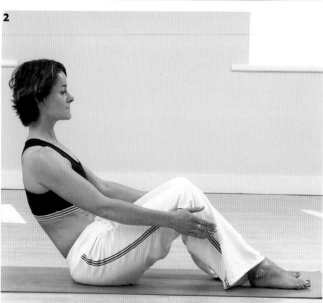

3

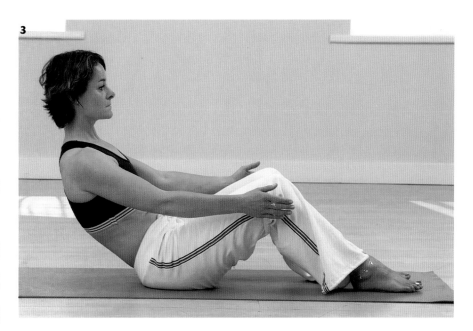

4

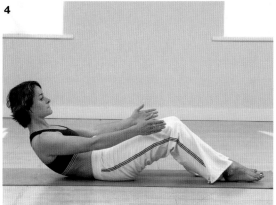

5

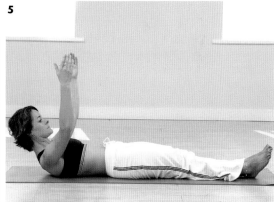

Hints & Tips

- Don't use momentum to get up off the floor, use control and strength.
- Maintain abdominal hollowing throughout the movement.

roll down (continued)

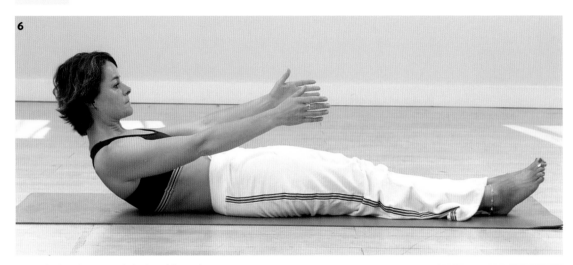

6 Slide the ribs toward the hip, lifting the head and shoulders and peeling the spine up off the floor, one vertebrae at a time.

7 Tilt the pelvis on the way up to get good segmental control.

8 Breathe out as you roll up and stretch toward the toes, sliding the shoulder blades back away from the ears, head between the arms. Bend the knees if needed.

9 Breathe in to start rolling back. Breathe out.

10 Maintain Transverse Abdominus and pelvic floor as you roll down toward the floor.

11 Finish with the arms back over the head, keeping the rib cage down.

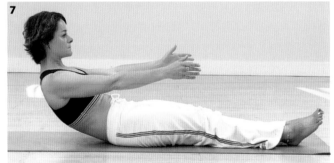

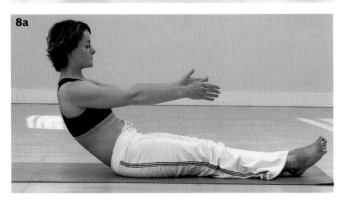

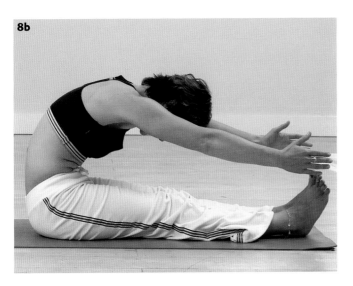

8b

Repetitions

- 5–10 times. The "c" curve and the abdominal preparation are good preparation exercises for this move.

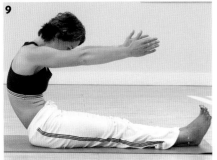

9

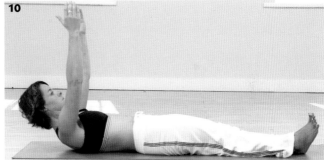

10

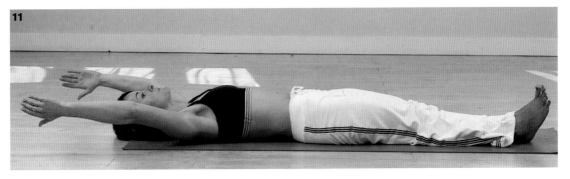

11

hamstring stretch
Beginner

Objectives: To lengthen the hamstrings, to develop core stability, and to strengthen trunk stability.

Start Position

- Supine position with one leg extended. Use an exercise band or long scarf around the extended leg.
- Shoulders relaxed and elbows down.

Technique

1 Breathe in to prepare.
2 Breathe out to engage Transverse Abdominus and pelvic floor and raise the leg slowly off the floor, maintaining neutral alignment in the spine and pelvis.
3 Breathe in and out for 3–5 breaths.
4 Breathe in.
5 Breathe out to engage Transverse Abdominus and pelvic floor and lower the leg to the floor.

Repetitions

- 3-5 on each leg.

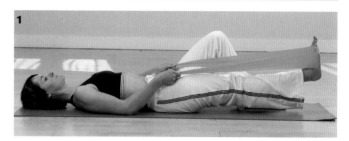

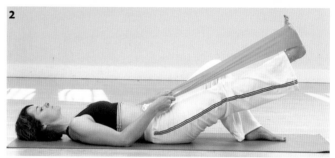

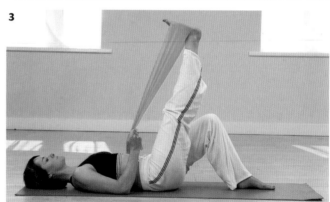

Hints & Tips

- Keep the pelvis in its neutral position.
- Keep the buttocks on the floor.
- Shoulders relaxed.
- Chin tucked slightly in to keep length in the back of the neck.

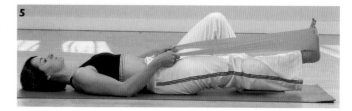

shoulder bridge
Intermediate

Objectives: Segmental control of the spine to increase mobility. To develop core strength. To strengthen gluteals and hamstrings. To strengthen trunk stability. To lengthen hip flexors.

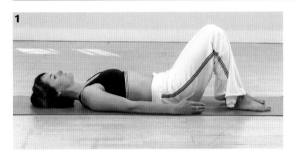

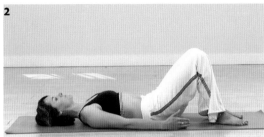

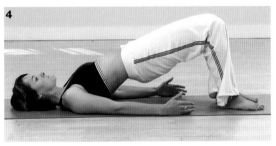

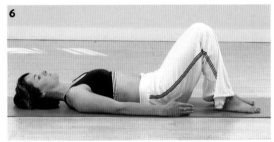

Start Position

• Supine set position—feet a little closer to the buttocks than you would normally.

• If you have been using a block under your head in this position, take it away for this exercise only.

Technique

1 Breathe in to prepare.

2 Breathe out, engage Transverse Abdominus and pelvic floor, and tilt the pelvis into imprint.

3 Breathe in.

4 Breathe out, maintain Transverse Abdominus and pelvic floor. Squeeze the buttocks and lift off the floor, peeling one verterbrae off at a time, lifting toward the shoulder blades.

5 Breathe in.

6 Breathe out, maintain Transverse Abdominus

and pelvic floor as you come down vertebrae by vertebrae, keeping the buttocks tight until they come back to the floor.

Repetitions

• Start with 5 and increase to 10.

Hints & Tips

• Keep checking that the abdominals are hollowed and the pelvic floor engaged.
• Check the weight distribution between your feet to see if you are favoring one side at any time.
• Only ever go up as high as comfortable.
• Don't allow the ribs to flare as you get higher off the floor.
• Keep knees in line during the lift.

129

hip roll
Beginner

Objectives: To mobilize the lumbar rotators of the spine. To strengthen the trunk stabilizers. To develop core strength. To strengthen the internal and external obliques.

Start Position

- The supine set position with your knees and feet together.

Technique

1 Breathe in to prepare.
2 Breathe out and engage the Transverse Abdominus and pelvic floor muscles.
3 Take the knees toward the right, turning the head toward the left.
4 Turn the left palm toward the floor to create stability in the shoulder leaving the right hand facing the ceiling.
5 Breathe in and hold.
6 Breathe out and engage the Transverse Abdominus and pelvic floor muscles and bring the knees and head back to center. Focus on using the obliques in the waist when returning to center.
7 Repeat to the other side.

Repetitions

- 5–10 times.

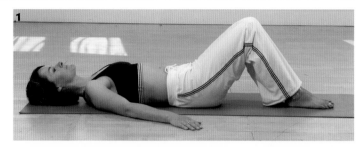

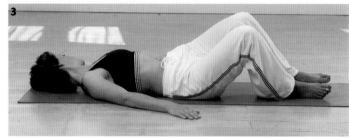

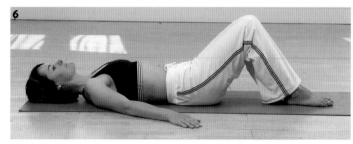

Hints & Tips
- Keep your shoulders down on the floor throughout.
- Don't take the legs too far to the side or the back will over extend, causing the ribs to rise.

hip roll
Intermediate

Objective: To lengthen and strengthen the obliques. To develop good rotation of the spine with segmental control. To promote awareness of the shoulder blades and to strengthen the shoulder stabilizers. Develops coordination ability.

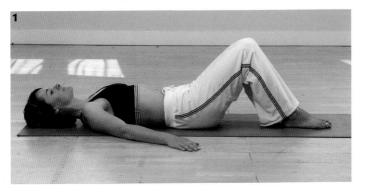

Start Position

- Start in the supine set position with your knees bent, arms at your side.

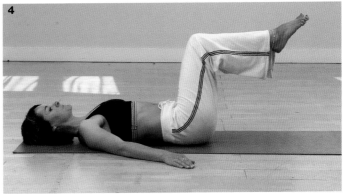

Technique

1 Breathe in to prepare.
2 Breathe out and engage the Transverse Abdominus and pelvic floor muscles to raise one leg off the floor.
3 Breathe in and imprint the spine by pressing the lower back gently toward the floor.
4 Breathe out and engage the Transverse Abdominus and pelvic floor muscles to raise the second leg without moving the spine.
5 Breathe in and hold.

131

hip roll (continued)

6 Breathe out, maintaining the engagement in the Transverse Abdominus and pelvic floor muscles, and take the knees to the left and turn the head to the right.

7 Breathe in and hold.

8 Breathe out, maintaining the engagement in the Transverse Abdominus and pelvic floor muscles, and return the legs and head to center.

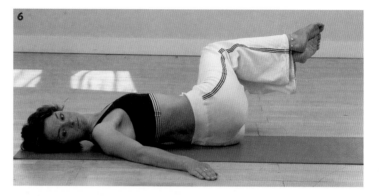

Repetitions

• 5 times on each side.

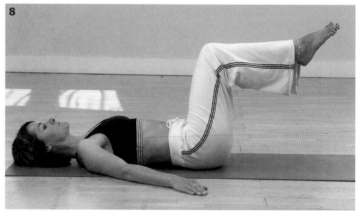

Hints & Tips

• During these exercises, be careful that the alignment is kept in the spine and in the neck. The alternate picture (right) shows how the alignment of the neck has been lost.

• Keep the awareness in the waist muscles which are initiating the movement on the return.

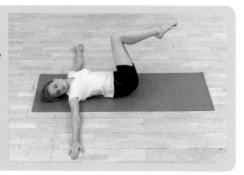

abdominal preparation
Beginner

This is a preparation exercise for lifting the head and shoulders off the floor.

Objectives: To strengthen the Transverse Abdominus while maintaining abdominal hollowing and lifting the head. Strengthening the core and shoulder stabilizers. Strengthening the deep neck flexors.

Start Position

- Start in the supine set position.

Technique

1 Breathe in to prepare.
2 Breathe out to engage the Transverse Abdominus and pelvic floor muscles.
3 Breathe in and drop your chin toward your chest.
4 Breathe out to slide the ribs toward the hips, hands toward the ankles.
5 Raise the head and the shoulders and look toward the knees.
6 Breathe in to return.
7 Breathe out to release and relax.

Repetitions

- Start with 5 and build up to 10 as it can be very tiring on the neck muscles.

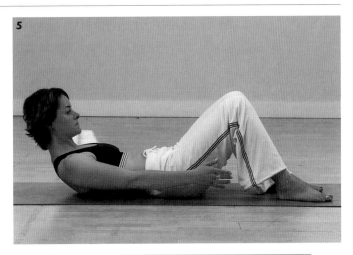

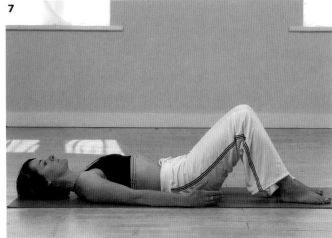

Hints & Tips

- Don't raise the head and shoulders if the abdominals are doming.
- Your buttocks stay relaxed.
- Pelvis stays in neutral.
- Don't forget to do the skull rock before lifting the head.

Modification:
- If you suffer with neck or shoulder problems do not lift head off the floor. Continue with everything else just omit the lifting of the head and shoulders.

133

side lying open door
Beginner

Objectives: To develop thoracic rotation. To strengthen shoulder stability. To stretch the chest muscle. To strengthen internal and external obliques.

Start Position

- Start in the side lying set position.
- Your feet are in line with your knees.
- Your knees in line with your hips.
- Your pelvis in its neutral position.
- Your rib cage is soft and down.
- Your shoulders are away from your ears.
- Your arms are out in front in line with your shoulders.
- Your shoulder blades are down.
- Tuck your chin in and keep your neck long.
- Breathe in and breathe out.
- Keep your pelvic floor engaged.

Technique

1 Breathe in to prepare.

2 Breathe out and engage the Transverse Abdominus and pelvic floor muscles and raise the arm toward the ceiling turning the head to follow the hand.

3 Breathe in to stay.

4 Breathe out to engage the Transverse Abdominus and pelvic floor muscles and close the arm following the hand with the head. The movement is in just the shoulder and head, and not the trunk.

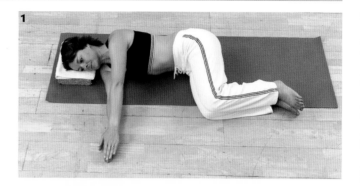

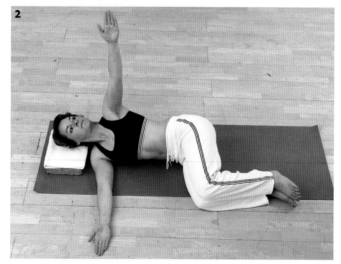

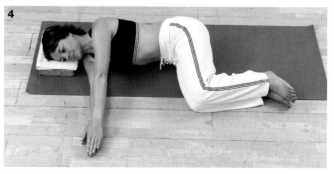

134

side lying open door
Intermediate

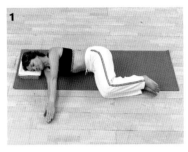
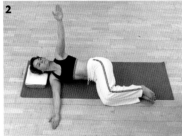
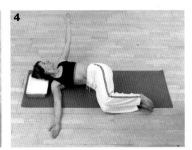

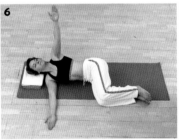
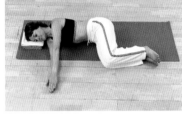

Start Position

- The side lying set position.

Technique

1 Breathe in to prepare.

2 Breathe out, engage the Transverse Abdominus and pelvic floor muscles and raise the arm toward the ceiling, turning the head to follow the hand.

3 Breathe in, hold the position, and stabilize the shoulder by dropping it toward the floor.

4 Breathe out, maintain the engagement in the Transverse Abdominus and pelvic floor muscles, and twist from the waist to open the chest. Follow the hand with the head, keeping the knees together and the hips stacked.

5 Breathe in and hold the position.

6 Breathe out, engage the Transverse Abdominus and pelvic floor muscles, and twist from the waist to return the body to its side position and point the arm toward the ceiling.

7 Continue to close the arm up.

Repetitions

- 5 is all that is required if done correctly. Repeat the movement on the other side.

Hints & Tips

- Keep your hips and knees together during the movement to keep the pelvis in alignment.
- If you have stiffness in the neck watch you only go as far as you can, keeping the nose in line.
- Initiate the twist from the waist (oblique muscle) in both directions, not from the shoulders.

135

swimming legs
Beginner

Objective: To strengthen the gluteals and hamstrings. To develop core strength. To lengthen the hip flexors.

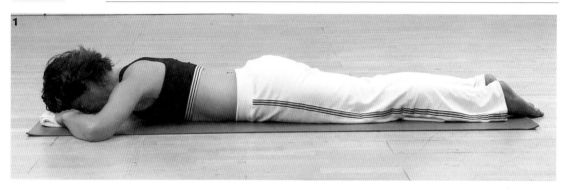

Start Position

- Start in the prone set position, supporting your head with your hands.
- Keep your feet apart in line with your knees.
- Your knees are in line with your hips.
- Your pelvis is in a neutral position.
- Engage the Transverse Abdominus muscles.
- Your rib cage is soft and down.
- Your shoulders are away from the ears, hands under the forehead.
- Your shoulder blades are down and engaged.
- Tuck your chin in to keep the neck long.
- Breathe in and breathe out.
- Engage the pelvic floor muscles.

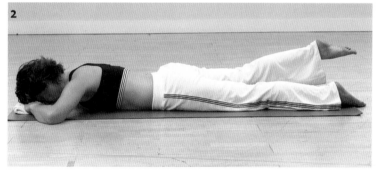

Technique

1 Breathe in to prepare.
2 Breathe out, engage the Transverse Abdominus and pelvic floor muscles, lengthen the legs, and raise one leg off the floor keeping the legs long.
3 Breathe in to return the leg to the floor.
4 Breathe out to engage the Transverse Abdominus and pelvic floor muscles, lengthen the legs and raise the other leg off the floor.
5 Breathe in to return the leg to the floor.

Repetitions

- 5 times with each leg.

Hints & Tips

- Keep both hip bones and the pubic bone on the floor as you lift the legs.
- Watch you don't tense up in the shoulders
- Don't bend the knees, keep lengthening away.

swimming arms
Intermediate

Objective: To develop coordination of upper and lower body. To strengthen shoulder stabilizers. To develop good scapula placement.

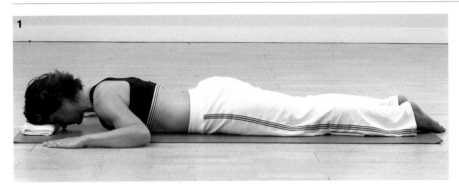

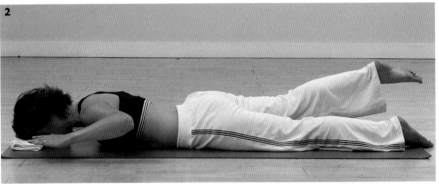

Start Position

- Start in the prone set position, with your arms in the "W" position (or with your arms by your side if the "W" causes tension in the shoulders).

Technique

1 Breathe in to prepare.

2 Breathe out, engage the Transverse Abdominus and pelvic floor muscles, and raise one leg off the floor, at the same time raising the opposite arm just off the floor, but not too high.

3 Breathe in to lower the leg and arm.

4 Breathe out, maintaining the engagement in the Transverse Abdominus and pelvic floor muscles, and raise the opposite arm to leg.

5 Breathe in to return.

Repetitions

- 5 times on each side.

Hints & Tips

- The movement of the arms is initiated by moving the spine.
- Bring the elbows back to the floor each time.
- If your elbows do not come to the floor, place the arms by your side.

swimming arms
Advanced

Start Position

• Start in the prone set position, with your arms in the "W" position (or with your arms by your side if the "W" causes tension in the shoulders).

Technique

1 Breathe in to prepare.

2 Breathe out and engage the Transverse Abdominus and pelvic floor muscles, sliding the shoulder blades down your back, raising the opposite arm to leg, and lifting the breast bone off the floor. Keep the head in alignment with the shoulders.

3 Breathe in to return.

4 Breathe out, maintain the engagement in the Transverse Abdominus and pelvic floor muscles, and lift the opposite arm to leg plus the breast bone.

5 Breathe in to return.

Repetitions

• 5 times on each side.

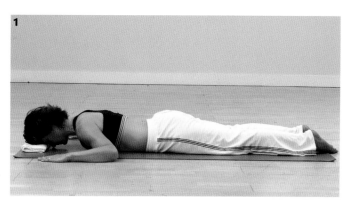

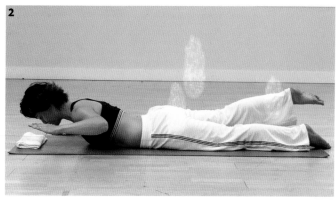

Hints & Tips

• Imagine you're holding a small peach under the chin, to assist in keeping head aligned.
• Don't be tempted to come up off the floor too high. Adding the breast bone lift is for thoracic extension only.
• Be sure to have practiced the breast stroke exercise before doing this progression.

Modification:
• At the end of the exercise, try doing a shell stretch to release the back. Stay in this position for a couple of breaths.

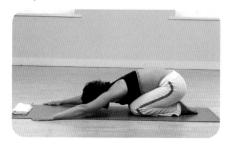

breast stroke
Beginner

Objective: To strengthen the postural muscles in the mid back for thoracic extension. To educate the scapula to fall into the correct placement. To strengthen the deep neck flexors.

Start Position

- Start in the prone set position. If you try this exercise and find you have an increase of pain or discomfort then do the first three steps of the exercise only and omit the lift of the breast bone.

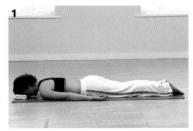
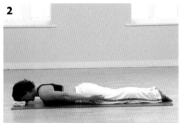

Technique

1 Breathe in to prepare.

2 Breathe out, engage the Transverse Abdominus and pelvic floor muscles, and draw the shoulder blades down and together. Raise the arms just off the floor externally rotating at the shoulder so the palms face one another. At this stage the head stays down.

3 If you have decided not to take this any further then release the shoulders back to the floor on an in breath, raising and stabilizing the arms in an out breath and repeating this 5–10 times. Make it an effortless movement.

4 Breathe in to slide the shoulder blades further down the back, raising the breast bone just off the floor, keeping the head in alignment with the shoulders, and maintain the engagement in the Transverse Abdominus muscles.

5 Breathe out to lower the breast bone to the floor.

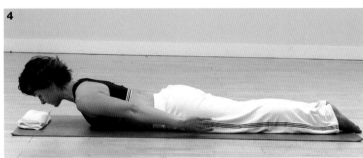

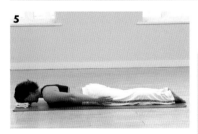

Repetitions

- 5-10 times.

Hints & Tips

- Watch that the head rest is not too high or too low. Your nose needs to be pointing down.
- Don't lift too high; the essence is on thoracic extension not lumbar.
- Keep the buttocks and legs relaxed. If you can't relax them, try placing the feet in the pigeon-toed position, which helps to disengage the activity in those areas.

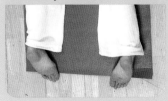

swan dive
Beginner

Objectives: To develop full spinal extension, to mobilize the lumbar spine, and to develop strength and stability in the shoulders.

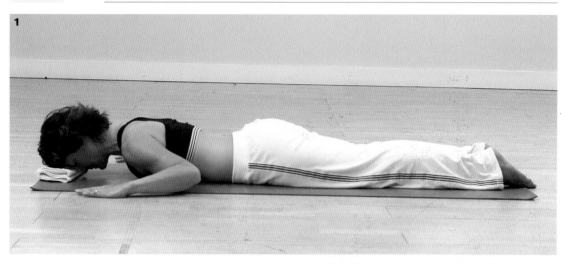

Start Position

- Start in the prone set position, with the arms in the "W" position.

Technique

1 Breathe in to prepare.

2 Breathe out, engage the Transverse Abdominus and pelvic floor muscles, slide the shoulder blades down the back, and raise the breast bone off the floor, keeping the elbows down.

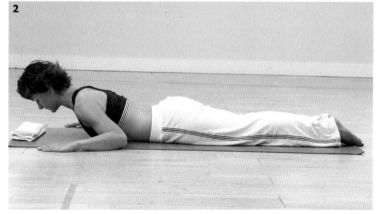

3 Breathe in to lift a little higher off the floor, raising the elbows, lengthening the arms, and extending the spine.

4 Breathe out, maintaining the engagement in the Transverse Abdominus and pelvic floor muscles, return onto the elbows. Keep your head up.

5 Breathe in, draw the shoulder blades down the back, and lift up through the spine.

Repetitions

- 5–10 times.

140

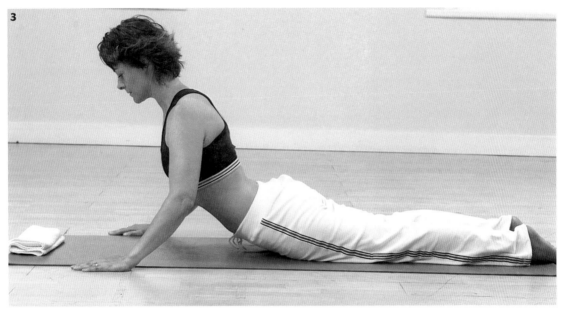

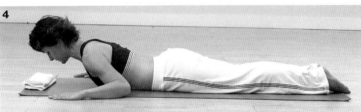

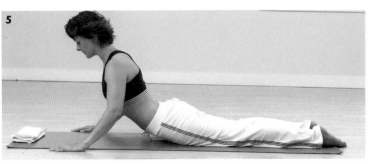

Hints & Tips

- Your elbows stay in toward the body and do not flare out.
- Your shoulders stay down away from the ears.
- Don't over extend or push higher than is comfortable.
- Keep your pubic bone down on the floor. The pictures actually show the pubic bone off the floor, which can happen easily if you have upper body strength but are inflexible in the lumbar spine. This is typical of the flatback posture, where the lower back is stiff.

141

cat's tail
Beginner

Objectives: To strengthen all trunk stabilizers focusing mainly on shoulder stability. To develop core strength. To strengthen the spinal extensors. To develop balance and strength.

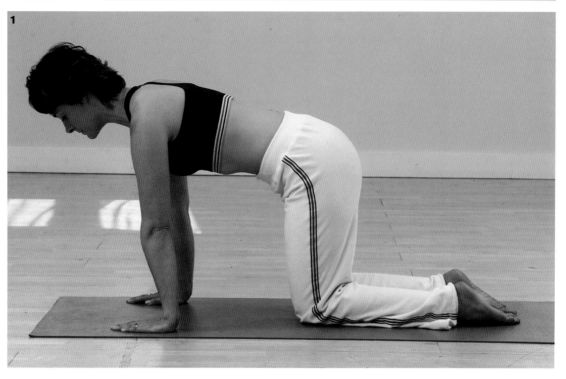

1

Start Position

- Start in the all fours set position.
- Your feet are apart in line with your knees.
- Your knees are in line with your hip bones.
- Your pelvis is in its neutral position.
- Engage the Transverse Abdominus muscles.
- Your rib cage is soft and down.
- Your shoulders are away from the ears and your hands are under the shoulders.

- Move your shoulder blades down your back.
- Tuck your chin in to keep the neck long.
- Breathe in and breathe out.
- The pelvic floor is engaged.

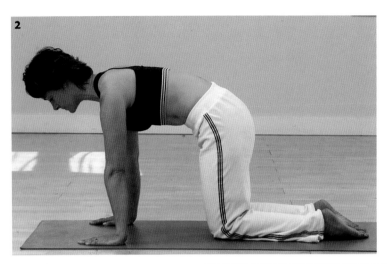

Technique

1 Breathe in to prepare.

2 Breathe out to engage the Transverse Abdominus and pelvic floor muscles, tucking the tail bone under (like a cat's tail going between its legs), and keeping the upper back stable and still.

3 Breathe in to return to the all fours set position.

Repetitions

• 5–10 times.

Hints & Tips

• This is far more difficult than you would think, especially with a flat back posture. If the lumbar spine is stiff you will round off in the upper back albeit unintentionally, this is because we have much more mobility in the thoracic spine than we do generally in the lumbar spine. Again, less is more.

• Maybe do this one alongside a mirror and watch your upper back.

• Placing a small ball on your upper back can help with the awareness of the movement. It will focus your attention straight away.

• Breathe in to sit back toward the heels into a shell stretch, after the movement (as below).

• Breathe out to relax and release. Give the hands a shake out.

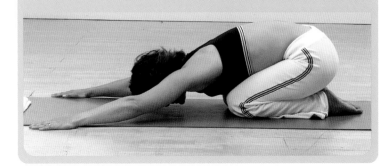

monkey squat
Beginner

Objectives: To develop correct lifting skills and strengthen trunk stabilizers while bending.

Start Position

• The standing set position.

Technique

1 Breathe in to prepare.

2 Breathe out, engage the Transverse Abdominus and pelvic floor muscles, and stabilize the shoulders. Hinge from the hips, taking the bottom back, and bending the knees.

3 Raise the arms to shoulder level, leading with the thumbs.

4 Breathe in to return to standing.

Repetitions

• Start with 5 and progress to 10.

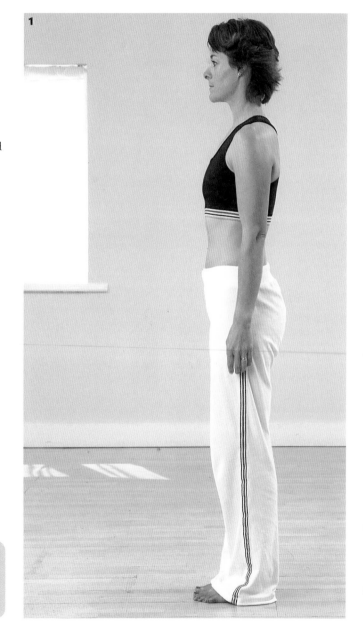

Hints & Tips

• Keep the spine in neutral alignment.
• Bend at the knees, not the waist.
• Keep the shoulders in line with the hips.

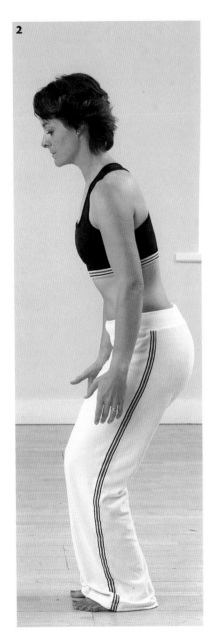

2

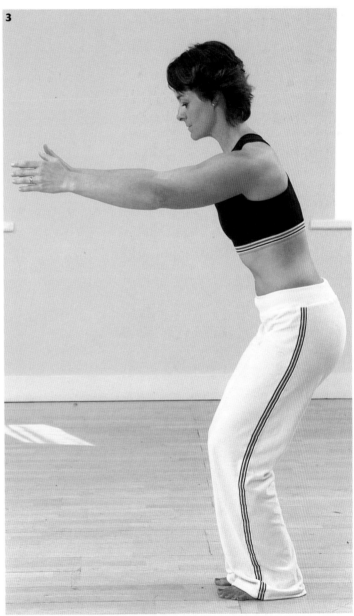

3

General Routine For Beginners

This short routine will help a beginner to start learning the principles in a way that will benefit all posture types. Through this routine, they can learn the ten commandments of Pilates and put them into practice.

heel slide
Beginner

Objective: To develop trunk stability. Mobility of the hip and stability in the pelvis to isolate the movement.

Start Position

- Start in the supine set position.
- Your feet are apart in line with your knees.
- Your knees are in line with your hip bones.
- Your pelvis is in its neutral position.
- Engage your Transverse Abdominus muscles.
- Your rib cage is soft and down.
- Your shoulders are away from the ears, arms by your side.
- Your shoulder blades are down.
- Tuck your chin in to keep the neck long.
- Breathe in and breathe out.
- The pelvic floor muscles are engaged.

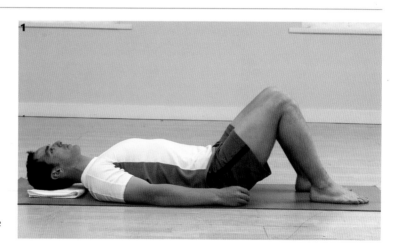

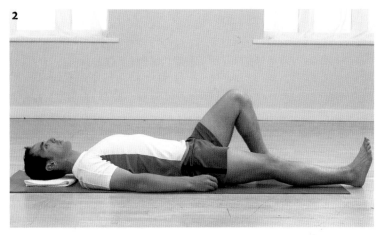

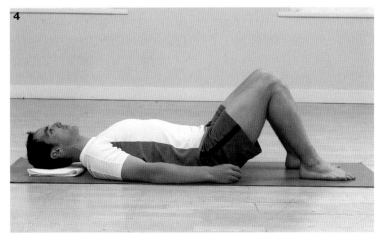

Technique

1 Breathe in to prepare.

2 Breathe out, engage the Transverse Abdominus and pelvic floor muscles and slide one leg away, maintaining pelvic stability.

3 Breathe in and hold.

4 Breathe out, engage the Transverse Abdominus and pelvic floor muscles, and slide the leg back to the set position.

5 Breathe in and hold.

6 Breathe out, engage the Transverse Abdominus and pelvic floor muscles, and slide the other leg away.

7 Breathe in and hold.

8 Breathe out, and engage the Transverse Abdominus and pelvic floor muscles, and slide the leg back to the set position.

Repetitions

• 5–10 times.

Hints & Tips

• Try using socks, if your feet are not sliding along the floor smoothly.
• Put your hands on hips if you want to detect movement.
• Keep it slow and don't rush your breathing—take time to feel what you're doing.

147

single arm pull over
Beginner

Objective: Helps trunk stability and to mobilize and stabilize the shoulder. Maintains correct rib cage placement.

Start Position

• Start in the supine set position.

Technique

1 Breathe in to prepare.

2 Breathe out, engage the Transverse Abdominus and pelvic floor muscles, and raise the arms toward the ceiling.

3 Maintain a neutral spine with your shoulders down and away from the ears, palms facing one another and chin tucked in.

4 Breathe in and hold.

5 Breathe out, engage the Transverse Abdominus and pelvic floor muscles, and take one arm slowly back toward the floor, leaving one arm pointing toward the ceiling.

6 Keep your rib cage down, don't let it flare.

7 Maintain a neutral pelvis, don't arch the back.

8 Keep your arms lengthened, don't bend at the elbows.

9 Breathe in to bring the arm back toward the ceiling.

10 Breathe out, engage the Transverse Abdominus and pelvic floor muscles, and take the other arm back.

Repetitions

• 5 times on each arm.

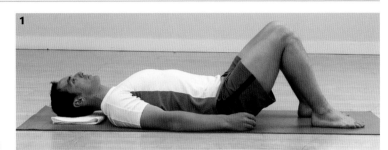

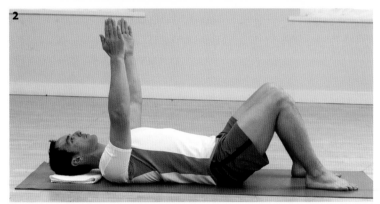

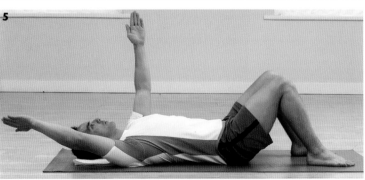

Hints & Tips

• You are not trying to touch the floor behind you.
• Keep your arms wide from the head.
• Your shoulders stay away from the ears.

seesaw arms
Beginner

Objective: Helps trunk stability and to mobilize and stabilize the shoulder. Maintains correct rib cage placement.

Start Position

- Start in the supine set position.

Technique

1 Breathe in to prepare.
2 Breathe out, engage the Transverse Abdominus and pelvic floor muscles, take one arm behind and one arm down by your side.
3 Breathe in to bring both arms back up to the ceiling.
4 Breathe out, engage the Transverse Abdominus and pelvic floor muscles, and take one arm behind and one arm down by your side.

Repetitions

- 5 times.

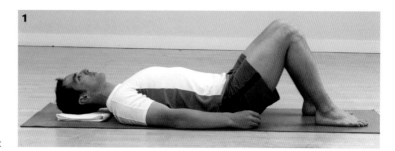

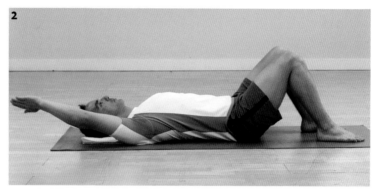

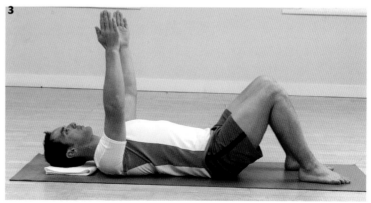

Hints & Tips

- Be very careful of the rib cage placement and twisting of the body during the movement.
- Keep your head stable and still on the floor.
- Maintain a neutral alignment.

Modification:
- You can also do a progression of this exercise by taking both arms behind the head together on the out breath, returning to the ceiling on the in breath.

149

heel slide and arm pullover
Beginner

Objective: To develop coordination skills on top of the stability factors.

Start Position

- Start in the supine set position with your knees bent and arms by your sides.

Technique

1 Breathe in to prepare.

2 Raise the arms toward the ceiling.

3 Breathe out, engage the Transverse Abdominus and pelvic floor muscles, slide one leg away, and (as in seesaw arms) take the opposite arm behind and the other arm down by your side.

4 Breathe in and hold.

5 Breathe out, engage the Transverse Abdominus and pelvic floor muscles, and bring the leg back and the arms back up toward the ceiling.

6 Breathe in and hold.

7 Breathe out, engage the Transverse Abdominus and pelvic floor muscles, and slide the other leg away using seesaw arms. The opposite arm to leg goes behind.

Repetitions

- 5 times.

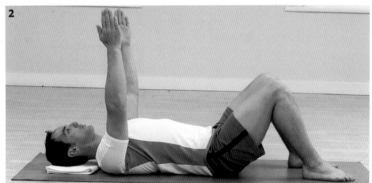

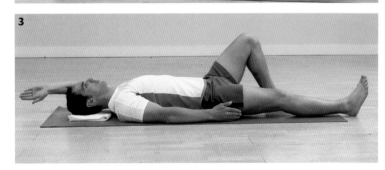

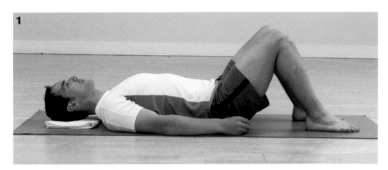

Hints & Tips

- Keep a neutral alignment.
- Watch the rib cage does not rise or the back arch.

double arm pullover and double heel slide
Beginner

Objectives: This exercise requires strong abdominal strength to prevent the spine from moving.

Start Position

- The supine set position.

Technique

1 Breathe in to prepare.
2 Raise the arms toward the ceiling.
3 Breathe out, engage the Transverse Abdominus and pelvic floor muscles to take both arms behind and to slide both legs away along the floor. Maintain a neutral spine.
4 Breathe in to raise the arms back toward the ceiling.
5 Breathe out, engage the Transverse Abdominus and pelvic floor muscles, slide the legs back in, and lower the arms back down by your side.

Repetitions

- 5–10 times.

Hints & Tips

- Use your breathing to assist in the movement.
- Keep your shoulders relaxed and your abdominals hollowed, especially on the return.
- Watch your back doesn't arch or imprint during the movements.

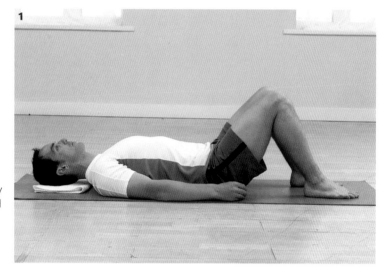

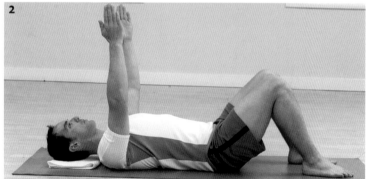

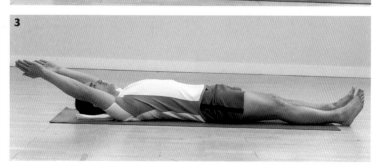

Extra Exercises

side plank level 1
Beginner

Objectives: To strengthen the abdominals, shoulder stabilizers, and shoulder girdle muscles.

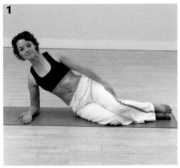 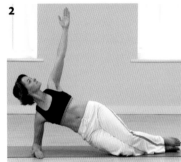 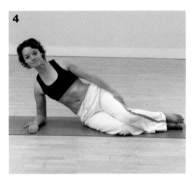

Start Position

- Start on your side, knees bent out in front, heels together, resting on the elbow, palms up. Your elbow is directly under the shoulder. Lift out of the arm so you are not slumping down.

Technique

1 Breathe in to prepare. Raise the top arm toward the ceiling and look up toward the hand.

2 Breathe out, engage the Transverse Abdominus and pelvic floor muscles, and lift the hips off the floor, reaching toward the ceiling.

3 Breathe in and hold.

4 Breathe out, maintain the engagement in the Transverse Abdominus and pelvic floor muscles, as you return to the floor.

Repetitions

- Initially repeat 3 times. As your stamina improves, aim to stay up in position for 3–5 breaths before returning to the floor to rest.

side plank level 2
Intermediate

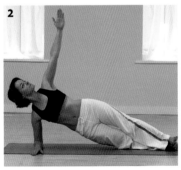

Start Position

- As in level 1, only with the legs outstretched, heels stacked.

Technique

1 Breathe in to prepare, raise the top arm toward the ceiling and look up toward the hand.

2 Breathe out, engage the Transverse Abdominus and pelvic floor muscles, and raise the hips.

3 Breathe in and hold.

4 Breathe out, maintain the engagement in the Transverse Abdominus and pelvic floor muscles, and return to the floor.

Repetitions

- Initially repeat 3 times. As your stamina improves, aim to stay up in position for 3–5 breaths, before returning to the floor to rest.

side plank level 3
Advanced

Start Position

- Sit to the side, resting on a hand, with the top leg open, and foot in front. Your back leg is bent at the knee, your foot sitting behind.

Technique

1 Breathe in to prepare and raise the top arm toward the ceiling.

2 Breathe out, engage the Transverse Abdominus and pelvic floor muscles, and push into the feet to lift off the floor, aiming the top hand toward the ceiling and lengthening the legs.

3 Breathe in and hold.

4 Breathe out, maintain the engagement in the Transverse Abdominus and pelvic floor muscles, bend the bottom knee to come back down to the floor.

Repetitions

- Initially repeat 3 times. As your stamina improves, aim to stay up in position for 3–5 breaths, before returning to the floor to rest.

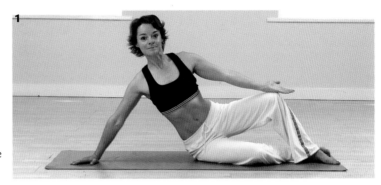

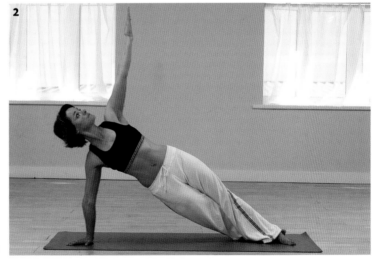

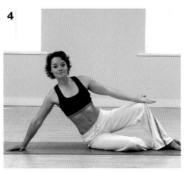

Hints & Tips

- Don't forget to do these side exercises on both sides.
- Keep the shoulder stabilized, while in up position.
- If your neck aches, look directly forward or to the floor until the neck muscles strengthen.

153

front plank level 1
Beginner

Objectives: To strengthen the abdominals and trunk stabilizers. Strengthen the gluteals and leg muscles.

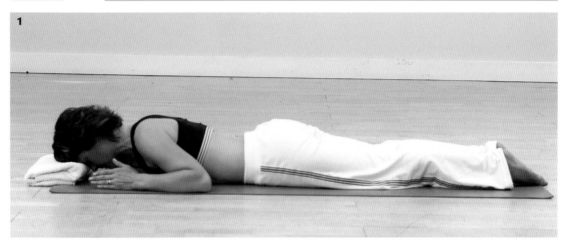

Start Position

- Start in the prone set position, with your arms tucked in, palms facing toward each other.

Technique

1 Breathe in to prepare.

2 Lift the breast bone and stabilize the shoulders.

3 Breathe out and engage the Transverse Abdominus and pelvic floor muscles.

4 Breathe in and hold.

5 Breathe out and return to the breast bone to the floor. Relax.

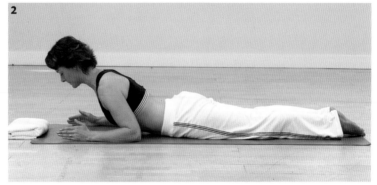

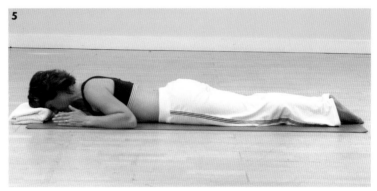

front plank level 2
Intermediate

Start Position

- Start in the prone set position, with your arms tucked in, palms facing toward each other.

Technique

1 Breathe in to prepare.
2 Breathe out, engage the Transverse Abdominus and pelvic floor muscles, stabilize the shoulders and start to raise the breast bone off the floor.
3 Continue to raise the breast bone.
4 Push up onto the knees, keeping the back aligned.
5 Breathe in and hold.
6 Breathe out, engage the Transverse Abdominus and pelvic floor muscles, and return to the floor to relax.

Repetitions

- Initially repeat 3 times. As your stamina improves, aim to stay up in position for 3–5 breaths.

Hints & Tips

- Keep the abdominals lifted.
- Don't round the back off. Keep the shoulder blades pulled in.
- Keep your hands facing up or toward one another.
- Don't clench the fists.

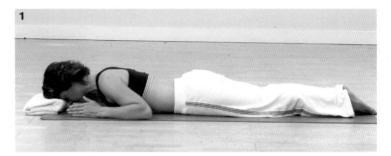

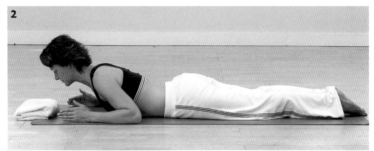

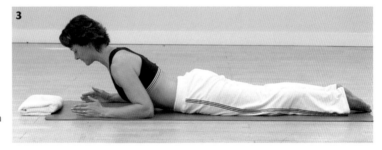

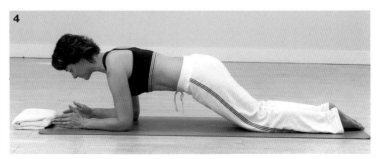

155

front plank level 3
Advanced

Start Position

- Start in the prone set position, with your arms tucked in, palms facing toward each other.

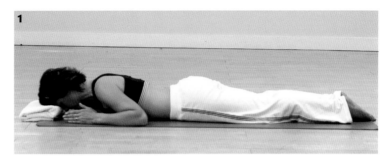

Technique

1. Breathe in to prepare.
2. Slide the shoulder blades down the back and raise the breast bone.
3. Continue to raise the breast bone.
4. Breathe out to engage the Transverse Abdominus and pelvic floor muscles, and squeeze the buttocks and the inner thighs together. Push into the balls of the feet and lift the body off the floor, keeping the spine level.
5. Breathe in and hold.
6. Breathe out and lower the body down to relax.

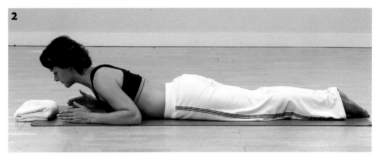

Repetitions

- Initially repeat 3 times. As your stamina improves, aim to stay up in position for 3-5 breaths.

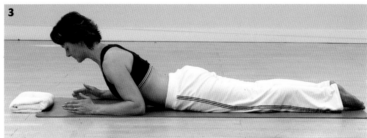

Hints & Tips:

- Don't raise the bottom higher than the shoulders.
- Watch yourself in the mirror.
- Don't clench the fists.
- Your weight should be distributed throughout the body not just in the shoulders.
- Keep your shoulder blades down and pulled in.

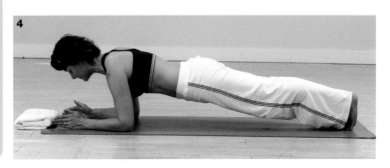

side leg lift part 1
Beginner

Objectives: To strengthen the muscles of the legs, to isolate the movement, and develop trunk stability while on the side.

Start Position

- Start in the side lying set position. If you have a problem getting the bottom arm to support your head, place a towel or block under the head and move the bottom arm out of the way.

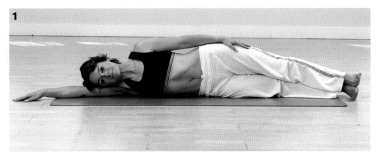

Technique

1. Breathe in to prepare.
2. Point the top toe away.
3. Breathe out, engage the Transverse Abdominus and pelvic floor muscles, and lengthen and lift the top leg.
4. Breathe in, hold, and flex the foot.
5. Breathe out, engage Transverse Abdominus and pelvic floor to lower the leg down.

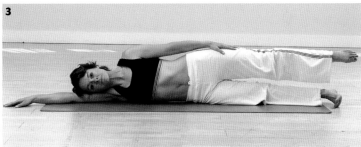

Repetitions

- 10 times.

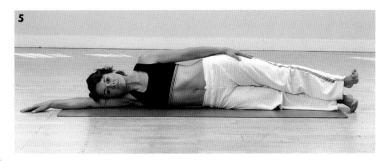

Hints & Tips

- If you are rolling back off the hips, place the top hand down in front of you for balance.
- Don't lift the leg too high, its about length not height.
- Keep the distance between the ribs and the hips when lifting the leg.

side leg lift part 2
Advanced

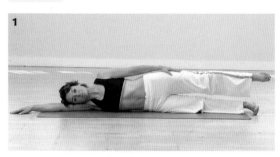

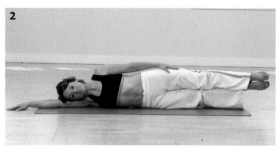

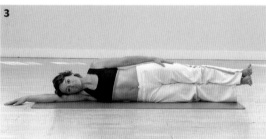

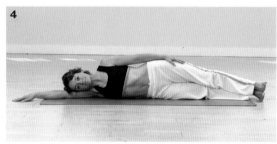

Start Position

- Start in the side lying set position. Use the top arm for balance.

Technique

1 Breathe in and point the top toe away, lifting the leg up slightly.

2 Breathe out, engage the Transverse Abdominus and pelvic floor muscles, and lift the bottom leg up to the top leg.

3 Breathe in and hold. Flex the feet.

4 Breathe out and lower the legs back down.

Repetitions

5–10 times.

Hints & Tips

- Keep the upper body relaxed.
- Use the top arm for balance but don't push into the supporting hand.
- Your head stays resting down.
- Bring ankle to ankle together, not toe to toe as seen below.

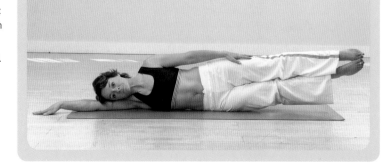

semi and full mermaid
Intermediate

Objective: To strengthen the Quadratus Lumbornum muscle, helping to keep correct alignment of the spine and pelvis. To develop balance and coordination.

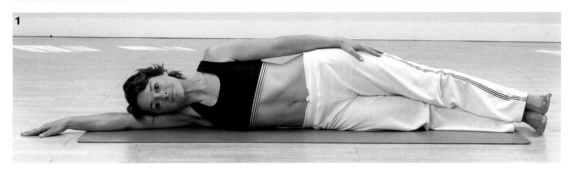

Start Position

- The side lying set position, with bottom arm extended up by ear.

Technique

1. Breathe in to prepare.
2. Breathe out, engage the Transverse Abdominus and pelvic floor muscles, hitch the top hip up toward the rib which will raise the legs off the floor.
3. Breathe in and hold.
4. Breathe out and release the hips back to lower the legs.
5. For the full mermaid draw the ribs down also to raise the upper body.

Repetitions

- 3–5 times.

Hints & Tips

- Keep the upper body relaxed.
- Initiate the move from the hips. Its not just a case of lifting the legs.

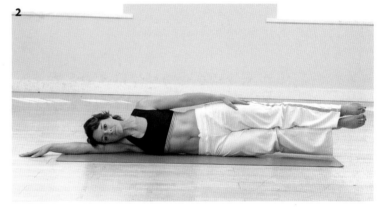

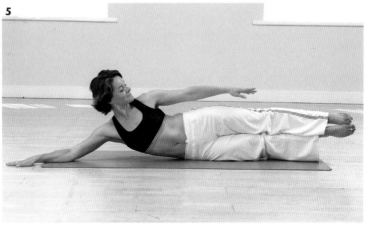

Index

Acknowledgments

All Images © Chrysalis Image Library/Mike Prior with the exception of the following;

Chrysalis Image Library:
© Chrysalis Image Library/Robyn Neild; 7.
© Chrysalis Image Library/Kuo Kang Chen; 10, 21

CORBIS: © Tim McGuire/CORBIS; 27

Chrysalis Books Group plc is committed to respecting the intellectual property rights of others. We have therefore taken all reasonable efforts to ensure that the reproduction of all content on these pages is done with the full consent of copyright owners. If you are aware of any unintentional omissions please contact the company directly so that any necessary corrections may be made for future editions.